The Patient's Internet Handbook

Dedications

To THK, MEK, GLK & JCA

The Patient's Internet Handbook

Robert Kiley BA (Hons), MSc, ALA
Head of Systems Strategy, Wellcome Library for the History and
Understanding of Medicine, Wellcome Trust

Elizabeth Graham MA, Dip Lib
Information Service Manager, Wellcome Library for the History and
Understanding of Medicine, Wellcome Trust

British Library Cataloguing in Publication Data
A catalogue record for this book is available from the British Library

ISBN: 1-85315-498-9

Typeset by Phoenix Photosetting, Chatham, Kent

Printed in Great Britain by Cromwell Press Ltd, Trowbridge, Wiltshire

For RSM Press
Commissioning Editor: Peter Richardson
Project Manager: Nora Naughton
Designer: Sarah Russell
Copy Editor: Miriam Richardson
Proof Reader: Joe Howarth
Indexer: June Morrison
Marketing Manager: Kirsty Orriss
Production Executive: Brian Weight

Table of Contents

Section 1 – Introduction and getting started

Section 2 – Searching for information

Section 3 – Your health and the Internet

Chapter 7 – NHS services and the Internet   93

Chapter 8 – Drug information on the Internet   105

Chapter 9 – Complementary and alternative medicine on the Internet   117

Section 5 – 100 medical conditions: sources of information on the Internet

About the authors

Robert Kiley is Head of Systems Strategy at the Wellcome Library for the History and Understanding of Medicine at the Wellcome Trust. He has written a number of related books including *Medical information on the Internet: a guide for health professionals* (Churchill Livingstone, 2nd edn, 1999) and the *Doctor's Internet Handbook* (RSM Press, 2000). He also edited the bi-monthly journal *He@lth Information on the Internet* from 1998 to 2000.

Kiley is a frequent commentator on health/Internet issues and has appeared on BBC Radio 4 and Sky Television.

Elizabeth Graham is Information Service Manager at the Wellcome Library for the History and Understanding of Medicine. She is an experienced Internet user and has run a number of training courses on how to search the Internet effectively.

Foreword

One of the consequences of presenting a TV programme called *Trust Me, I'm a Doctor* is that people fail to spot the irony and ask 'Why?'. Or, as one critic put it, 'A better title would be *Trust Me, You Have No Choice*'. True, in an emergency there isn't much else you can do other than lie back and have blind trust in whatever the NHS has to offer you, but in most other situations you do have a choice. You can accept what you're told as Gospel, or you can check for yourself whether you've been given the best advice or offered the best treatment.

Although Britain is the most secretive of all the Western democracies and has traditionally relied on blind faith in experts, the Internet looks set to change all that. Of course, if you log onto a consumer health site you may just be swapping the opinion of your own doctor with the opinion of a cyberdoc, and it can be very hard to judge who's right. Or worse still, you may end up with fraudulent or flakey advice from someone with no qualifications whatsoever, whose only aim is to sell you an 'amazing miracle cure'.

Swapping blind trust in doctors for blind trust in the Internet would be disastrous, and what we need is an expert guide to steer us away from the snake oil salesman and towards legitimate sites offering help and support based on the best available evidence. This is where *The Patient's Internet Handbook* can help. It's meticulously researched, well written and so useful that within a week of reading it, it's helped me do a better job as a journalist, a doctor, a teacher and a patient. This isn't to say you should spend all day surfing the net – I can't think of anything more unhealthy – but when you need fast access to reliable health information, this book is the place to start.

No book or Internet site can replace a consultation with a doctor, but it will help you go in there as an equal and get the most out of your meeting. This may mean you have to think more about the choices offered to you and deal with more uncertainty, but there is clear evidence that patients who are informed and involved in decisions about their health do better. And now there's no excuse not to.

Dr Phil Hammond
GP, lecturer, writer and broadcaster and adviser to <http://www.pocketdoctor.co.uk>

Preface

The Internet is changing the way we live and work. E-mail is rapidly becoming the communication medium of choice, whilst the Web provides the opportunity to access a range of services at the click of a mouse. Services such as Internet shopping and banking – virtually unheard of two or three years ago – are now mainstream activities.

The Internet, however, offers far more than a convenient place to shop and conduct business. For the information-seeker the Internet gives access to a wealth of resources, far greater than any library can ever hope to provide. In the field of medicine and health, key information sources – such as medical databases, textbooks, clinical guidelines and drug compendiums – can now be accessed by anyone who has a connection to the Internet. Before the development of the Internet much of this information was only available to doctors and other health professionals.

As access to the Internet has become more prevalent – figures from the Office of National Statistics show that 37% of UK households can connect to this network – so more people are using it to find information about health and disease. One recent study from the US reported that some 56% of US citizens who have Internet access use it to find health information. This figure is greater than the percentage of people who shop online or use the Internet for investment information.

The purpose of this book is to introduce you to the wealth of health information on the Internet and explain, through examples, how you can find health information specific to *your* needs. With this information you can become more informed about your health and play a more active role in the health care process. Being informed, however, does not make us into doctors, surgeons or diagnosticians! It is important that information found on the Internet is taken to the consulting room where its suitability and appropriateness can be fully evaluated by a health professional.

To provide a clear navigational structure to this book we have divided the contents into five discrete sections. Section 1 takes the form of an introduction and gives practical advice on how to connect to, and use, the Internet. Section 2 builds on these skills and considers how you can find health information that is accurate, timely and appropriate. Section 3 adopts a more subject-focused approach and looks at what information and services you can access through the Internet. Throughout the book attention is paid to the quality of health information on the Internet and section 4 examines this issue and provides guidance on how to evaluate the information you find. The final section takes the form of a directory of Web-based information sources for 100 common medical conditions.

The size and volatility of the Internet means that any book on this topic can never be anything more than a snapshot of what is available. New resources appear and, more frustratingly, established ones change or simply disappear in the void of cyberspace.

To help minimise the frustration this causes, many of the Web sites discussed and referenced in this book can be accessed from *The Patient's Internet Handbook* Web site <http://www.patient-handbook.co.uk>. If we become aware that a site has moved we will endeavour to find its new location and publish its new address on this Web site.

You can also use this site to contact the authors with any questions you have about the book, or to suggest items or topics for inclusion in any future edition.

Robert Kiley & Elizabeth Graham
July 2001

Acknowledgements

We would both like to thank the many people – most of whom we only met in cyberspace – who took the trouble to respond to our information requests.

We would especially like to thank Peter Richardson (Director of RSM Press) for his unfailing support throughout this project and Genevieve Kiley for the work she performed in proofreading the text.

Robert Kiley & Elizabeth Graham
July 2001

Introduction and getting started

Overview

The purpose of this book is to introduce you to the wealth of health information on the Internet, and explain, through examples, how you can find health information specific to *your* needs. With this information, you can become more informed about your health and play a more active role in the healthcare process.

In this introductory section – Chapters 1 to 3 – we provide an overview of health information on the Internet and consider what you need to be able to access and exploit this information.

Chapter 1 highlights the range of health information and help available on the Internet and gives an overview of this book as a whole, along with some useful introductory tips. Chapter 2 discusses what you will need to get connected to the Internet and provides guidance on how to choose an Internet Service Provider (ISP). Once you are connected to the Internet you need to know how to make effective use of e-mail and the Web browser. This is the theme of Chapter 3, where, in addition to providing a guide to these tools the chapter also considers more advanced features, such as configuring your browser to filter out undesirable content and how to encrypt your e-mail to ensure that it cannot be accessed by anyone other than the intended recipient(s).

CHAPTER 1

Consumer health information on the Internet

Introduction

In matters pertaining to health few people subscribe to the view that 'ignorance is bliss'. On learning that we, or a close friend or relative, are suffering from a particular medical condition one of the first things we do is try to find some more information about the illness. Typically, we want to know if it is life threatening, is there a cure, does any treatment have side effects, and what is the long-term prognosis?

In finding answers to these questions, your doctor is *always* the best person to ask. Indeed, only he/she is aware of your specific circumstances and medical history. At the same time, however, many of us feel the need to seek out additional information. The motivational factors behind this are varied. Perhaps we feel the doctor has not the time to explain all we need to know, or there are questions we feel we cannot ask through fear or embarrassment. Equally, we may wish to find additional information so we can ask meaningful questions and understand the treatment options. In trying to satisfy these needs most people turn to their local library hoping that they can find some relevant literature, or perhaps be put in touch with a local support group.

In the past couple of years, however, the development and widespread availability of the Internet have transformed access to health information. Information on *any* matter relating to health is now never more than a few mouse-clicks away. To give a few random examples, you can use the Internet to:

- learn how to conduct an effective breast self-examination <http://www.drkoop.com/family/womens/breast/bse.asp>;
- identify the health risks of holidaying in West Africa (Fig. 1.1) <http://www.fitfortravel.scot.nhs.uk/>;
- understand the relative risks pertaining to measles, mumps, rubella (MMR) vaccine <http://www.immunisation.org.uk>;

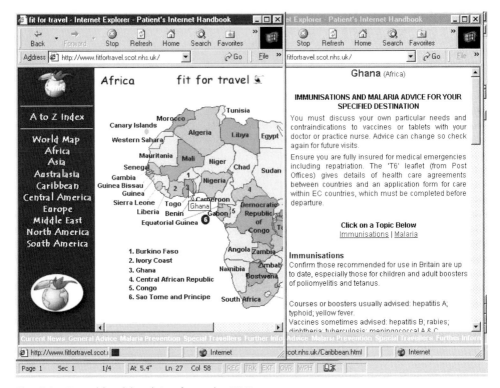

Fig. 1.1   Travel health advice from the NHS

- learn, through interactive tutorials, what happens during heart surgery (Fig. 1.2)
  <http://www.nlm.nih.gov/medlineplus/tutorials/coronaryarterybypass-graft.html>;
- discover the latest evidence-based research on a range of health topics
  <http://www.cochraneconsumer.com/>;
- identify waiting times information for your local NHS hospital
  <http://www.doh.gov.uk/waitingtimes/>.

In addition to giving access to information, the Internet also provides the opportunity for health consumers to communicate with fellow patients (and health professionals) throughout the world. This can be especially valuable if you are caring for someone with a relatively rare condition where the chances of meeting up with anyone in a similar position may be somewhat limited.

Purpose of this book

The purpose of this book is to introduce you to the wealth of health informa-tion on the Internet, and explain, through examples, how you can find health

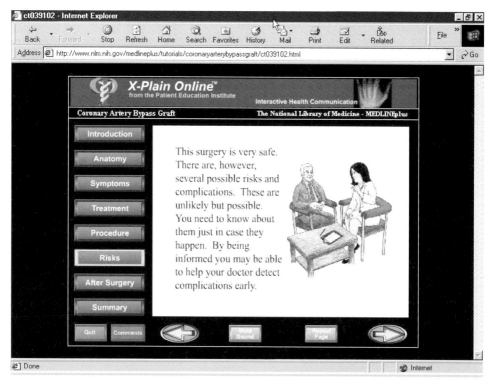

This surgery is very safe. There are, however, several possible risks and complications. These are unlikely but possible. You need to know about them just in case they happen. By being informed you may be able to help your doctor detect complications early.

Fig. 1.2   Heart surgery – interactive tutorials

information specific to *your* needs. With this information, you can become more informed about your health and play a more active role in the healthcare process. Indeed, research shows that people who participate in decisions about their treatment experience less anxiety and may have improved health outcomes.

Right from the start, however, it should be made clear that the Internet should not be used as some form of surrogate doctor. Though the Internet helps all of us become more informed about our health, it does not turn us into diagnosticians, pharmacists or surgeons. Information we find on the Internet should be brought to the consulting room where its suitability can be fully discussed and evaluated.

Using this book

To provide a clear navigational structure to the book we have divided the contents into five discrete sections. Though the book can be read from cover to cover, it is also possible to dip into just those sections that are most relevant to the reader.

Section 1 – Introduction and getting started

This section provides an introduction to health information on the Internet, along with advice on how to connect to the Web (Chapter 2) and guidance on how to use the key Internet software tools, namely the Web browser and e-mail (Chapter 3). These chapters will be useful both to new Internet users (or those thinking about getting connected to the Internet) as well as to more experienced users, who will find information on topics such as broadband access and configuring your browser to filter out undesirable content.

Section 2 – Searching for information

These next three chapters focus on how you can find health information specific to your needs. Chapter 4 looks at the different types of Internet search tools – search engines, Web directories, and evaluated gateways – and provides examples and analysis of how these tools can be used most effectively. Chapter 5 takes the concept of searching a stage further and looks at the premier medical databases – used by today's health professionals – that everyone can now access via the Web. Specifically, this chapter provides a practical guide to searching MEDLINE, Cochrane Database of Systematic Reviews and the Complementary and Alternative Medicine Citation Index.

The last chapter in this section (Chapter 6) introduces the reader to Internet discussions lists and newsgroups and provides tips and advice on how you can find discussion forums relevant to your interests.

Section 3 –Your health and the Internet

In this section we look at a number of health topics and discuss the range of information and services health consumers can obtain via the Internet.

For most people the NHS is the sole provider of health care and in Chapter 7 we consider to what extent the NHS has embraced the Internet and discuss what information the consumer can obtain via this medium. Specifically, we examine the availability of waiting times and performance data and consider what additional information is required before patients can become truly empowered.

Drug information is the focus of Chapter 8, where in addition to giving an overview of the key information sources, we discuss the rise of the online pharmacy and the potential dangers it poses.

Interest in complementary and alternative medicine (CAM) is massive and in Chapter 9 we provide a guide to the key CAM resources on the Internet.

The final chapter in this section looks at the information sources on the Internet pertaining to pregnancy, childbirth and infant care. Topics covered include tests and scans, giving birth, and immunisation, as well as providing information about a number of interactive tools such as an ovulation calculator and an online birth plan.

Section 4 – Keeping safe

Throughout the book attention is paid to the quality of health information that is published on the Internet. As the Internet enables *anyone* to publish *anything* we need to adopt a healthy scepticism to the information we find. Chapter 11 looks at the quality issue and discusses practical ways in which we can protect ourselves from dubious Web sites.

Chapter 12 brings together all the themes covered in the book and considers to what extent the Internet has led to the rise of the empowered patient. The chapter includes information on how best to prepare for the consultation and to present to your doctor information found on the Internet.

The final chapter in this section looks to the future and the possible role the Internet will play in the delivery of health care.

Section 5 – 100 medical conditions: sources of information on the Internet

The final section takes the form of a directory presenting information about support groups, online discussion lists and newsgroups. For each subject discussed we highlight a number of introductory documents, published by trustworthy sources, which can be accessed via the Web.

Accessing Internet resources

Throughout this book we provide references to numerous Web sites. To access any of these sites open up your Web browser and key-in the Web address (known as the URL, or Uniform Resource Locator) as cited. Thus, using an example from above, to find the latest official information on the MMR vaccine you can enter the following URL: <http://www.immunisation.org.uk>. Note, however, that you should **not** input the chevrons <> that prefix and suffix every URL. These are included to separate the URLs from the main body of the text.

Alternatively, many of the Web sites discussed in this book can be accessed from the Patient's Internet Handbook Web site at <http://www.patient-handbook.co.uk>. This site will also be used to alert readers to any changes in the URLs published in this book. You can also mail the authors with any questions you have about the book or suggest items for inclusion in any future edition.

Conclusion

A recent survey conducted by the Pew Internet and American Life Project concluded that 56% of US citizens who had access to the Internet used it to find health information. Even more striking is the fact that this figure is greater than the percentage of people who shop online or use the Internet to find investment information. Though no comparable figures are readily available in the UK, figures from the NHS Direct Online service show that in the first four weeks of operation the site attracted over seven million hits. These figures clearly demonstrate the high level of interest in online health information.

This book will show you – the healthcare consumer – how to search the Internet effectively and exploit the resources that are now available. With this knowledge at our fingertips we all have the opportunity to become informed and active participants in the healthcare process.

Connecting to the Internet

Introduction

Until a few years ago the task of connecting a computer to the Internet was highly complicated and one that was best left to computer whizz-kids. Indeed, paediatrician Tim David, in a letter to the *British Medical Journal* in 1996, remarked that 'only serious computer enthusiasts with plenty of spare time should access the Internet from home'.

In the years that have passed since this letter was published the task of connecting to the Internet has been significantly simplified. Anyone who can install a computer game or a piece of office software has the necessary skills to connect a computer to the Internet. At the same time, however, the connection choices available to the home user – dial-up access, cable modems, ADSL, unmetered calls etc – have multiplied. The purpose of this chapter is to explain, in a non-technical way, the options available and to highlight the issues that need to be considered before you hook your computer up to the Internet.

In this chapter we will assume that access to the Internet will be made via a computer. If you wish to access Internet services through your television set – thus avoiding the need to invest in a personal computer – please note that a number of companies, such as NTL and OnDigital, provide this service. Contact these companies directly for more information.

Getting started

To connect to the Internet you need the following components:

- A computer
- Software – networking software, plus a Web browser and an e-mail program
- A modem and telephone line
- Internet Service Provider (ISP)

Up and running in 10 minutes

Assuming that you have a computer, a modem and a telephone line the easiest way to connect to the Internet is to acquire a 'Getting connected' CD-ROM, freely available from numerous high street stores (Dixons, Tesco, Boots etc), as well as banks, building societies and even garages. These CDs contain all the software you need to connect to the Internet, plus an installation program to help configure your computer. Once the installation program has been run, connecting to the Internet should be no more difficult than opening up any other application (word processing program, games etc) on your computer.

Though for many the task of configuring and connecting will stop at this point, it is still worthwhile to look in more detail at the individual components that make up the Internet connection. In particular, you may wish to change your Internet Service Provider (ISP) (or set up access to many providers thus minimising the likelihood of ever being denied access by an engaged dialling tone), or consider moving to broadband, high-speed access.

Computer

Almost any computer, of any specification, can be connected to the Internet. However, to enjoy the full multimedia capabilities of the Internet – video clips, audio files etc – the recommended minimum specification is a computer with a Pentium processor and 32 megabytes of memory. A CD-ROM drive is also very useful as most ISPs (discussed below) supply their 'getting connected' programs on CDs. Any new computer will vastly exceed these minimal requirements.

Software

To make the actual connection to the Internet, software programs are required to dial your chosen ISP and to enable your computer to 'talk' to other computers. One reason why the Internet is so universal is that all the connected computers – irrespective of whether they are a Windows-based PC, an Apple Mac, or a Unix machine – speak the same language. For the technically minded the international computer language is TCP/IP (Transmission Control Protocol/Internet Protocol). Fortunately, you do not need to know anything about these protocols to use the Internet.

Once a connection has been made you need a Web browser to read pages on the Web, and an e-mail program to send and collect messages. Details on how to use these applications are discussed in Chapter 3.

All the software programs discussed here will either already be on your computer, or will be supplied free of charge by your ISP.

Modem

A modem is required to connect the computer to a data transmission line, typically a telephone line. Indeed, until fairly recently it was the only means by which the home user could connect to the Internet. A modem, using analogue telephone lines devised in the nineteenth century, is always going to be relatively slow, and as the Internet has become more multimedia in format, the call for faster access has been ever greater. Over the past 12 months this call has been met (albeit slowly) with the introduction of cable and ADSL (Asymmetric Digital Subscriber Line) modems.

Your decision on whether to purchase a traditional modem or a much faster cable or ADSL modem will depend first and foremost on whether the high-speed alternatives are available in your locality. If cable television is not readily available then the cable modem option is a non-starter. Equally, if your local British Telecom exchange does not yet support ADSL you will not be able to take advantage of this technology. To determine whether your BT exchange has been ADSL-enabled visit the ADSL Availability Checker at: <http://www.pipex.net/adsl/availability.shtml#popup> (Fig. 2.1).

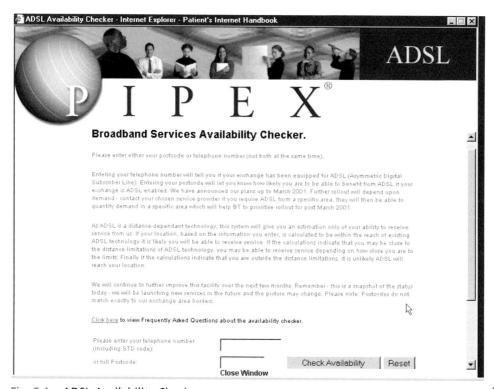

Fig. 2.1   ADSL Availability Checker

Table 2.1   Dial-up and broadband access: some comparisons

	Costs	Advantages	Disadvantages
Dial-up	• 56k modem £60.00 • No set up or installation costs • Pay-as-you-go phone charges or unmetered access	• Easy to get connected • Available everywhere	• Relatively slow • Analogue lines subject to line noise – Web pages may need to be re-requested
ADSL	• Modem & installation fee of £150.00 • Monthly subscription – average cost £50.00	• High-speed access • No call charges – connection is 'always on' • Can still make telephone calls whilst online – no need for a 2nd line	• Limited availability. At launch only 26% of UK homes could access an ADSL-enabled exchange • Even if your exchange is enabled, to make use of this technology you need to live no further than 2.5 miles from the exchange • New technology – expect teething problems
Cable	• Cable modem & installation fee – £175.00 • Monthly subscription – £40.00	• High-speed access • No call charges – connection is 'always on'	• Only available in cable franchised areas

Assuming these technologies are available in your locality you still need to ensure that your ISP allows you to access their services via these methods. Finally, you need to consider whether the additional hardware costs (modems that support high-speed access are more expensive than the traditional dial-up modem) are worth paying.

For further information on broadband access and how this compares with the traditional dial-up access, see Table 2.1.

Internet Service Provider

The final piece of the connection jigsaw is the Internet Service Provider. Each ISP has a permanent connection to the Internet, which you log into as and when you need access to Internet services. Via your ISP you are able to access the Web, transfer files and send and receive e-mails. Almost certainly, your ISP will also provide you with free Web space you can use to create your own Web pages.

When you have finished accessing these services you log out. However, as the ISP remains online at all times any mail sent to you when you are not connected is received and held. When you next connect, the mail is downloaded to your computer.

As of March 2001 there are in excess of 300 ISPs in the UK. The majority of these providers offer a subscription-free access route to the Internet. All you will be liable for is the call charge (levied by your phone company) to connect to the ISP. In all cases this will be charged at local call rates.

In addition to these subscription-free services, ISPs are also beginning to offer unmetered dial-up access – you simply pay a fixed monthly fee irrespective of how much use you make of the Internet – and high-speed access using broadband technologies.

Choosing your ISP

With so many ISPs, all offering a broad spectrum of access options, picking the best one is far from straightforward. For example, though the subscription-free services may appear to be the best option (how can you argue with something that costs nothing?) you may find that the helpdesk support from these providers is very expensive. If you are new to the Internet and think that you may require this type of support, the free services may prove to be expensive!

To help select the ISP that addresses your needs most closely, the following questions should be considered:

1. What does your existing phone company offer in terms of Internet access?

The major UK telecommunication companies were initially very slow in providing Internet access to their customers. Issue three of the *.Net Internet Magazine* (February 1995) provided a review of 'every major British ISP'. The list comprised just 20 service providers – amongst which the telecommunication companies were conspicuous only by their absence.

Times have now changed and the two leading UK phone companies – BT and NTL – offer a variety of Internet access packages. Before signing up with any other ISP it is worth checking to see what is available from these companies as existing customers may be able to benefit from special offers.

2. How much use are you likely to make of the Internet?

If you are only likely to make occasional use of the Internet – perhaps for sending e-mail and the occasional foray on the Web – then the

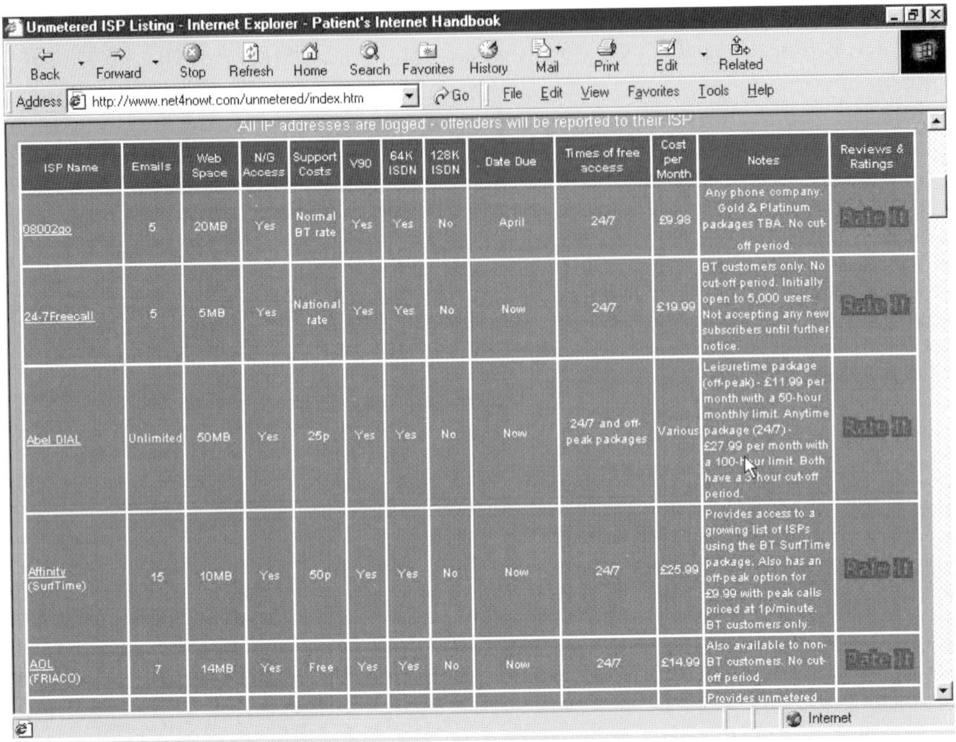

Unmetered ISP Listing - Internet Explorer - Patient's Internet Handbook

Address http://www.net4nowt.com/unmetered/index.htm

All IP addresses are logged - offenders will be reported to their ISP

ISP Name	Emails	Web Space	N/G Access	Support Costs	V90	64K ISDN	128K ISDN	Date Due	Times of free access	Cost per Month	Notes	Reviews & Ratings
08002go	5	20MB	Yes	Normal BT rate	Yes	Yes	No	April	24/7	£9.98	Any phone company. Gold & Platinum packages TBA. No cut-off period.	Rate It
24-7Freecall	5	5MB	Yes	National rate	Yes	Yes	No	Now	24/7	£19.99	BT customers only. No cut-off period. Initially open to 5,000 users. Not accepting any new subscribers until further notice.	Rate It
Abel DIAL	Unlimited	50MB	Yes	25p	Yes	Yes	No	Now	24/7 and off-peak packages	Various	Leisuretime package (off-peak) - £11.99 per month with a 50-hour monthly limit. Anytime package (24/7) - £27.99 per month with a 100-hour limit. Both have a 3-hour cut-off period.	Rate It
Affinity (SurfTime)	15	10MB	Yes	50p	Yes	Yes	No	Now	24/7	£25.99	Provides access to a growing list of ISPs using the BT SurfTime package. Also has an off-peak option for £9.99 with peak calls priced at 1p/minute. BT customers only.	Rate It
AOL (FRIACO)	7	14MB	Yes	Free	Yes	Yes	No	Now	24/7	£14.99	Also available to non-BT customers. No cut-off period.	Rate It
											Provides unmetered	

Fig. 2.2 Details of unmetered access ISPs at the Net4Nowt site

subscription-free Internet service providers, such as Freeserve or Virgin, will be more than adequate.

If your Internet use increases – and you find that you are paying in excess of £10.00 per month on Internet call charges – then it would be cost effective to move to one of the unmetered access providers. An up-to-date listing of all UK ISPs offering unmetered access can be found at: <http://www.net4nowt.com/unmetered/index.htm> (Fig. 2.2).

3. How important is fast access?

If you connect to the Internet through a standard dial-up modem the fastest access speeds you will enjoy will be 56 kbps. This is adequate for sending and receiving mail and for most Web browsing. This form of access, however, will appear very slow when accessing Web sites that make heavy use of multimedia technologies, such as video clips and sound files, or if you download large software programs. On a dial-up 56k modem Microsoft estimate that it takes more than two hours to download a copy of their Web browser.

To mitigate such problems you may wish to consider using an ISP that supports access via broadband technologies such as ADSL and Cable modems. These technologies will allow download speeds from the Internet at up to 8Mbps – some 140 times faster than a 56k modem. Note, however, that though these speeds are technically possible most ISPs offer customers connection speeds of between 512 kbps and 2Mbs. Even so these speeds still represent somewhere between 9 and 35 times faster than a 56k modem.

Broadband technologies also allow you to make voice calls at the same time as you are online – thus avoiding the need for a second telephone line. Finally, as this technology is 'always on' (there is never any need to log on – you are permanently connected to the Internet) there is never any delay in receiving or sending e-mails.

An up-to-date listing of all UK ISPs offering broadband access can be found at: <http://www.net4nowt.com/broadband/index.htm>.

4. What sort of support will you need?

To help recover some of the costs involved in providing subscription-free Internet access, a number of ISPs provide technical support via premium rate telephone lines. In such cases the call costs are in the order of £1.00 a minute. Consequently, if telephone support is a key requirement then using one of the subscription-based ISPs may prove to be cost effective. For example, customers who subscribe to the basic America OnLine (AOL) service (£9.99 a month) get support via a free-phone number.

5. Do you need 'roaming' services?

If you do a lot of international travelling and wish to be able to access the Internet in precisely the same way as you do at home it makes sense to sign up with an ISP that has international points of presence (POPs). AOL, for example, has POPs in more than 185 countries. For users of this service the Internet is rarely more than a local phone call away.

6. What are you prepared to pay?

Though fast access speeds with toll-free support lines may be the preferred solution the costs may be prohibitive. The average monthly ISP subscription fee for broadband access is around £40.00 for 512 kbps access. Higher speeds will incur even greater costs. In contrast the subscription-free services attract no costs, other than those incurred by dialling the ISP.

ISPs – further information

Table 2.2 provides brief details on some of the leading UK ISPs. For the very latest information see the Net4Nowt site at: <http://www.net4nowt.com/>. If

Table 2.2   Leading UK ISPs

Name	Web address	Free dial-up	Subscription dial-up	Unmetered	ADSL	Cable	Contact
AOL	\<http://www.aol.com\>	✗	✓	✓	✗	✗	0800 376 5432
BT Internet	\<http://www.btinternet.com\>	✓	✓	✓	✓	✗	0800 800 001
Demon	\<http://www.demon.net\>	✗	✓	✓	✓	✗	0845 272 2999
Freeserve	\<http://www.freeserve.net\>	✓	✗	✓	✓	✗	0879 500 049
IC24	\<http://www.ic24.net\>	✓	✗	✓	✓	✗	09067 444 222
Madasafish	\<http://www.madasafish.net\>	✓	✗	✓	✓	✗	0870 050 0333
Ntl	\<http://www.ntl.co.uk\>	✓	✗	✓	✗	✓	0800 052 1815
Pipex Dial	\<http://uk.uu.net\>	✗	✓	✓	✓	✗	0870 600 4454
Virgin	\<http://www.virgin.net\>	✓	✗	✗	✗	✗	0500 558 8000
World Online	\<http://www.worldonline.co.uk\>	✓	✓	✓	✗	✗	0800 542 1717

you do not have access to the Internet, the *Internet Magazine* (published monthly) provides a regular guide to UK ISPs and publishes results of bench-mark tests detailing how each ISP has performed over the past month.

Conclusion

As this chapter has demonstrated, connecting to the Internet is relatively straightforward and can be achieved without incurring significant costs. Indeed, leaving aside the investment in the computer and modem, costs are fairly minimal, and if you opt for unmetered access, completely predictable. In contrast, the wealth of information available through the Internet is both staggering and, in terms of value, unquantifiable.

Before we consider how we can find and exploit this information, however, we need to examine briefly how we use the key Internet tools – namely the Web browser and e-mail. This is dealt with in Chapter 3.

The Web browser and e-mail

Introduction

A recent survey of Internet connectivity concluded that around 380 million people now have access to this medium. Though this figure clearly shows that the Internet is not quite as pervasive as we sometimes assume – the world's population is estimated to stand at 6 billion – when access is examined at a more regional level we see the massive impact the Internet has made in developed countries. In the US some 53% of the population are connected whilst in the UK figures from the Office of National Statistics show that around 35% of UK households have access to the Internet.

Though part of this growth in connectivity can be ascribed to curiosity and a wish not be left behind in the information revolution, repeated surveys on *why* individuals are connecting to the Internet shows two recurring (and obvious) themes. First, there is a desire to access the Web, and through this to gain access to information resources as well as services, such as online shopping and banking. The second is a wish to communicate cheaply and easily with friends and colleagues throughout the world. To achieve this, e-mail is recognised as the communication tool of choice.

In this chapter we will discuss these services – the Web and e-mail – focusing in particular on how to make effective use of the software to access these services. Details on how to find information on the Web is dealt with in Chapters 4 and 5, whilst guidance on the use of e-mail in the health context – how you can communicate with fellow patients and carers etc – is the subject of Chapter 6.

The Web browser

The development of the Web browser revolutionised the way the Internet was used and subsequently evolved. Prior to its development, Internet services could only be accessed through character-based software (no pointing and

Table 3.1   Web browsers – supporting applications

Application	Purpose, cost and availability
Adobe Acrobat	Many Web sites contain files in a pdf (portable document format) style. Documents published in this format have exactly the same 'look and feel' as an original paper version. Fonts, layout, pagination etc are all retained. PDF files can only be viewed – not edited. Cost: Free Available at: <http://www.adobe.com>
Internet Explorer	Microsoft's Web browser Cost: Free Available at: <http://www.microsoft.com>
Netscape Navigator	Netscape's Web browser Cost: Free Available at: <http://www.netscape.com>
QuickTime	A number of sites – such as CNN – distribute videos in a QuickTime format. To view such videos QuickTime software is required. Cost: Free Available at: <http://www.apple.com/quicktime>
Real Player	A number of sites – such as BBC Online – publish videos in a Real Player format. To view such videos Real Player software is required. Cost: Free Available at: <http://www.real.com>
Telnet	Though the character-based interface that goes with Telnet looks somewhat dated after the slick sophistication of the Web, there are still some sites that can only be accessed by Telnet. A wide number of Telnet programs are available, many of which can be accessed from the TUCOWS site. Cost: Free Available at: <http://www.tucows.com/>

clicking). Because this form of access was not particularly easy to use it did not attract a mass-market audience, which in turn limited the development of Internet services. In 1993, however, the first graphical Web browser was released (known as Mosaic), and the rest, as they say, is history.

The Web browser was the 'killer application' the Internet was looking for. Suddenly, Internet services could be accessed at a mouse-click, and more importantly, related resources could be linked through the use of hypertext. Hypertext allows you to move from one resource to another – even if they happen to be on opposite sides of the world – at the click of a mouse.

Although today there are a number of Web browsers available, the market is dominated by Netscape's Navigator and Microsoft's Internet Explorer. Both are available free of charge and can be acquired either on CD-ROM (distributed by ISPs or magazines that focus on the Internet) or directly from the Internet.

In addition to being able to display Web pages, browsers can be used to download files, and plug-in to related applications. For example, video clips on the Internet are usually distributed in either a QuickTime or Real Player format, whilst many official publications are in a PDF format. Though the browser cannot by default handle these media formats, if you have the appropriate software programs, your browser can be configured to open these applications. Once this has been done all files can be seamlessly accessed through one piece of software – the Web browser. Table 3.1 provides details of the most popular Internet plug-ins, along with details of how they can be obtained.

Using the browser – the basics

Irrespective of which browser you use, all support common features that can be accessed through the standard toolbar (Fig. 3.1). Table 3.2 provides a summary of these features.

It is worth noting that when using the Web you can simultaneously open up multiple browser windows. Thus, if one site appears to be responding very slowly, you can leave that browser window running in the background and open another window to access another site and continue working. Dependent upon how much memory your computer has you can typically have at least four browser windows running at once without any serious impact on performance. New windows can be opened by the keystroke Ctrl-N. (Hold down the Control key (Ctrl) and press the letter N.)

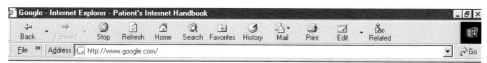

Fig. 3.1   The Internet Explorer toolbar

Table 3.2   Web browser – toolbar functions

In the following table, function commands appear in the form **menu name** ◊ **command**. Thus, **File** ◊ **Save**, means open the file menu and select the save option.

Ctrl refers to the Control key, located at the bottom left-hand side of the keyboard.

Where commands are browser specific IE will be used to indicate Internet Explorer and NS to signify Netscape's Navigator.

Toolbar option	Function
Back & Forward	Use these keys to go back (and forward) to Web pages previously accessed.
Stop	Use to stop loading the current page – a useful function if the page is big (in terms of the number of images etc) and/or slow.
Refresh	Sometimes a page will be corrupted as it is transmitted. This will be evident in either missing text or images. Using the Refresh key forces the browser to go back to the original server and re-request the page.
Home	The Home page is the page the browser defaults to when the application is first opened. This should be set to open up the page *you* consider to be most useful. A search engine, or medical database (Chapters 4 and 5) may be a suitable candidate. IE – **Tools** ◊ **Internet Options** ◊ **General** ◊ **Home Page** NS – **Edit** ◊ **Preferences** ◊ **Navigator** ◊ **Home Page**
Search	Use this button to connect to an Internet search engine. See Chapter 4 for details.
Address/Location	This is where the Web address (known as a URL) of every page is displayed. This address/location box can also be used to enter the address of any Web page you wish to access. Throughout this book you will see Web addresses in the form <http://webaddress.suffix>. If you want to access any of these pages simply enter the full address as cited in the address/location box. If you prefer, the http:// prefix can be omitted.
History	The History function can be used to view offline previously accessed pages. IE – **File** ◊ **Work Offline**. Click on the History icon (or press **Ctrl-H**) NS – **File** ◊ **Offline** ◊ **Work Offline**, then **Communicator** ◊ **Tools** ◊ **History** (or press **Ctrl-H**) Any page in the History file can be selected and viewed.
Multiple windows	Use **Ctrl-N** to open up multiple browser windows.

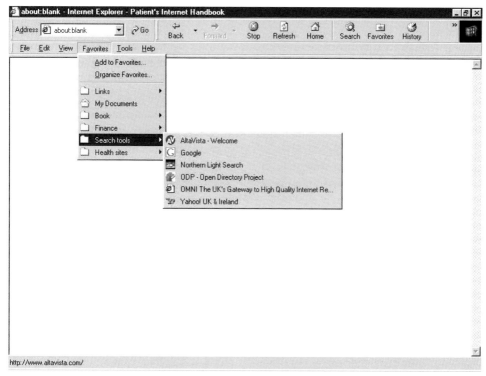

Fig. 3.2   Bookmarks – arranged hierarchically for easy access

Bookmarks and favourites

As you start to explore the Internet there will undoubtedly be some sites you will wish to return to. MEDLINE (Chapter 5), for example, is a key resource that anyone interested in current medical research will need to access on a regular basis. Though you can re-key the Web address <http://www.ncbi.nlm.nih.gov/PubMed> every time you wish to access this site, it makes more sense to use the Bookmark/Favorite feature within the Web browser to record this (and other) URLs. (Netscape uses the term Bookmarks whilst Microsoft prefers Favorites.)

Once a site has been 'bookmarked' subsequent visits to that resource can be made by calling up the bookmarked list and clicking on the relevant site (Fig. 3.2). As the list of favourite sites grows you may wish to consider organising these into subject-specific folders to facilitate easy access.

Saving Web pages

If you are connected to the Internet via a pay-as-you-go telephone service it makes sense to save text-heavy Web pages on your computer and read them offline, away from the ever intrusive ticking of the online call-charging clock.

In the more recent versions of these browsers (Internet Explorer version 4.0 and above; Netscape Navigator 4.75 and above) every Web page you access in any Web session is saved to your hard disk. To access this store of pages, known as the cache, you need to instruct the browser to work offline (otherwise, the browser will continue to try and connect to the Internet) and open up the history file.

Typically, pages in the cache are arranged by date. Web pages will remain accessible via the history file until the pages are deleted or until the amount of space taken up by these pages reach a predetermined maximum size. These settings can be changed using the **Preferences** menu.

If you are not using a browser that supports automatic saving, pages can still be stored using the **File** ◊ **Save as** option. However, this is a far more cumbersome method and upgrading your browser may be a more effective option.

Security

There has been a great deal of concern about whether it is safe to conduct business over the Internet – in particular is it wise to transmit your credit card details? Though any system is open to abuse, if the Web sites you are accessing

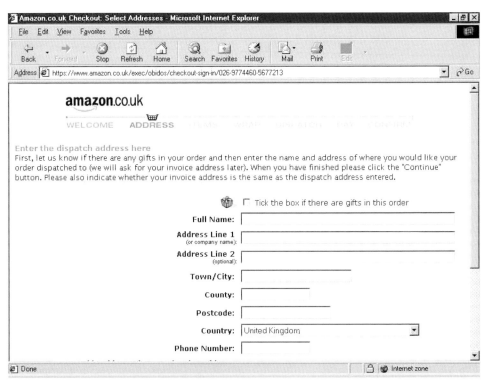

Fig. 3.3   Secure page as seen through Internet Explorer – note the locked padlock

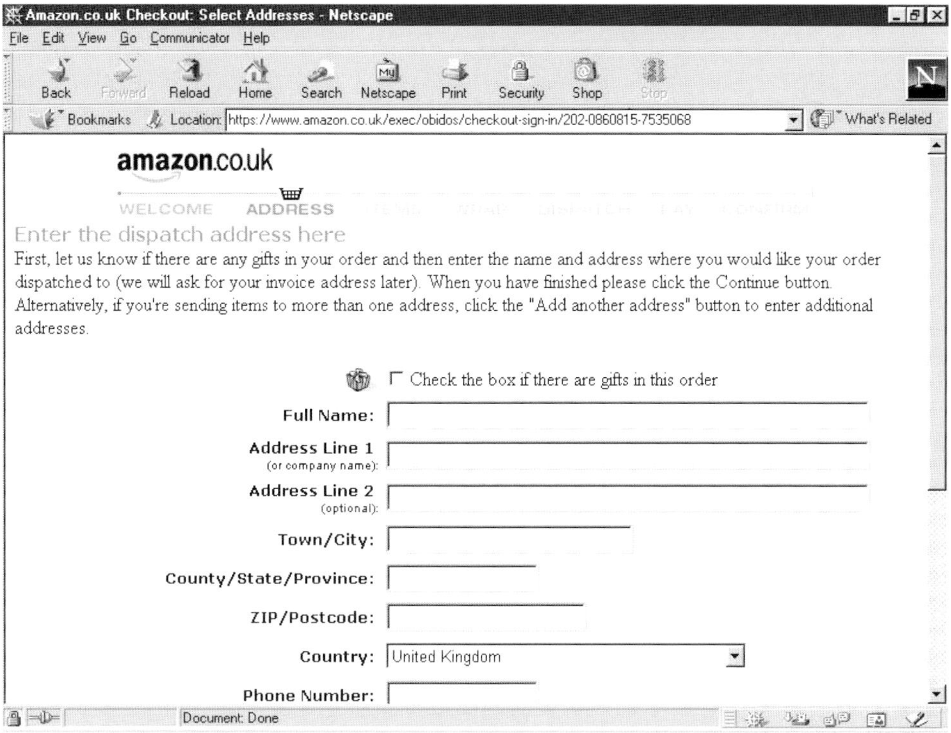

Fig. 3.4 Secure page as seen through Navigator – note the locked padlock

use a secure system you can be reasonably assured that your transaction will not be tampered with.

When accessing a secure site users of Internet Explorer will be presented with a dialogue box informing them of this change in status (by default Web pages are not secure) and a locked padlock will appear on the bottom of the browser window (Fig. 3.3). Navigator users will be presented with a similar alert, along with a symbol of a locked padlock (Fig. 3.4).

Filtering content

There may be occasions when you want to filter the information that can be found on the Internet. For example, the easy availability of pornography on the Internet is well known and if children are going to use the Internet it is advisable to introduce some form of filtering.

Though you can download various content-filtering software programs from the Internet, both the leading browsers have in-built filtering facilities which filter material based on agreed international standards (PICS or Platform for Internet Content Selection) and personal preferences.

The mechanism behind content filtering is very simple. At the browser level

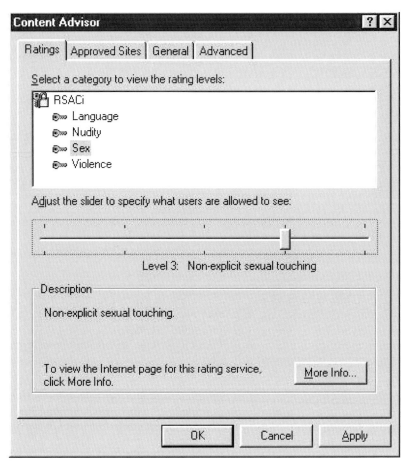

Fig. 3.5   Defining the level of filtering in Internet Explorer

you determine the level of filtering you wish to employ (Fig. 3.5). At the other end of the chain, Web authors embed tags into a Web page to indicate the level of nudity or violence on a specific page. More advanced tagging systems – such as that developed by Safe Surf – allow authors to use tags based on themes such as drug abuse and gambling. Once the level of filtering has been defined, access to any Web page whose content exceeds that level is denied. Box 3.1 describes how content filtering can be enabled using Internet Explorer and Netscape Navigator.

Obviously there are many Web pages that contain material that is unsuitable for viewing by children but do not contain PICS tags. One solution to this is to set up your filtering profile to exclude every page that has not been rated. However, in doing this you will be denied access to many useful sites, simply because the author has not rated them.

A number of organisations have drawn up codes of practice for 'safe browsing' and parents interested in this topic are advised to read the one

Box 3.1   Filtering content

Internet Explorer

- In Internet Explorer content filter is enabled by clicking on: **Tools** ◊ **Internet Options** ◊ **Content** ◊ **Content Advisor** ◊ **Enable**

Through the 'Enable' tab you can specify the level of language, nudity, sex and violence on which you wish to filter. The violence tab, for example, has four levels ranging from Level 0 'No violence', through to Level 4 which is defined as 'Wanton and gratuitous violence'.

- Once the levels have been enabled you are prompted for a supervisor password. Using this prevents other users from changing or disabling these settings.
- If at any point you wish to change the filtering levels click on: **Tools** ◊ **Internet Options** ◊ **Content** ◊ **Content Advisor** ◊ **Settings**.
- By default, once the content advisor has been enabled, pages that have not been rated cannot be seen. To disable this somewhat draconian approach click on: **Tools** ◊ **Internet Options** ◊ **Content** ◊ **Content Advisor** ◊ **Settings**. In the **Content Advisor** Tab click on **General** and make sure the option 'Users can see sites that have no rating' is checked.

Navigator

Setting up content-filtering in Navigator is achieved by completing a Web-based form on the Netscape Web site.

- Connect to the Internet and then click on **Help** ◊ **Netwatch**. When the resulting page is loaded follow the link to **NetWatch Setup process**.

NetWatch allows you to define levels of filtering for two rating scales: RSACi (the one recognised by default by Internet Explorer) and the more sophisticated SafeSurf ratings. Simply select which (or both) of these you wish to use and the level of filtering you want to employ. For example, the SafeSurf Rating scheme has rating scales for specific subjects, such as gambling and drug abuse. Taking the latter case, you can opt to filter sites at Level 0 (blocks all sites that have been rated as 'Glorifying drug abuse') through to Level 9 where only those sites that 'Solicit Personal Participation' in drug abuse are blocked.

- When you are happy that the correct level of filtering has been enabled, make sure the **NetWatch On** radio button is checked and then follow the link to **Save Changes**. At this point you will be prompted to define a password, which ensures that your filters cannot be altered.
- If you want to be able to see unrated sites, ensure that the 'Allow users to see unrated sites' is checked.

developed by the Internet Watch Foundation, available at: <http://www.internetwatch.org.uk/safe/tip.htm>.

E-mail

Despite the attention that is afforded to the Web, the desire to be able to send and receive e-mails is often the key motivating factor for seeking Internet access. E-mail is fast, virtually cost-free and highly efficient (Box 3.2). It can be used to send both text and binary files (word-processing files, spreadsheets, images etc.); and once you start using it in earnest, the idea of writing and posting a letter (now known as snail mail) or sending a fax seems somewhat labour intensive!

E-mail – the basics

To send and receive e-mails you require e-mail software. As mentioned earlier, this will typically be provided free of charge by your ISP. If this is not the case (or if you want to use a different program) a range of e-mail programs can be downloaded from: <http://dmoz.org/Computers/Software/Internet/Clients/Mail/>.

Box 3.2   Advantages of e-mail

Fast
In practice most e-mails reach their destination within a few minutes of being sent. The exact time depends on how many mail servers (which work in the same way as post office exchanges) any single message has to be routed through, and how busy the network is. In the unlikely event that a message takes in excess of four hours your local mail server will usually send you an e-mail alerting you to this and informing you that it will continue trying to deliver the message.

Cheap
Unlike telephone calls and the postal service where costs are related to the location that you are trying to reach, all e-mails are treated equally. It costs no more to send a message to Birmingham, Alabama than it does to send the same message to Birmingham, UK.

Efficient
As long as a message is correctly addressed you can, for the most part, be assured that the message will reach the recipient. If you do cite an invalid mail address the message will be returned.

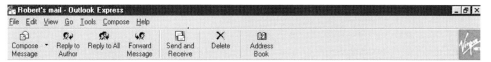

Fig. 3.6   Outlook Express (e-mail) toolbar

Irrespective of which e-mail program you use, all support common features that can be accessed through the standard toolbar (Fig. 3.6). Table 3.3 provides a summary of these features.

Table 3.3   E-mail – toolbar functions

Toolbar option	Function
Compose message	Opens up a new window for you to compose your e-mail.
To; cc; Bcc	In this box you enter the e-mail address of the person you wish to communicate with. Via the *cc* option you can copy the message to another person or group of people. *Bcc* (blind carbon copy) allows you to copy the message to a third party (or groups of people) without the original recipients (as identified in to *To*: section) being aware of this.
Reply/ Reply to all	One of the powerful and attractive features of e-mail is that you can reply to any message by a single keystroke. You do not need to bother about keying in an e-mail address – the e-mail software will do that for you – and as the original message is included in the reply, answers can be inserted immediately adjacent to any question. If a message had been copied to others, the *Reply to All* option will send your one response to all recipients.
Forward	Use this option to forward any received e-mail to anyone else you think might be interested in it.
Address book	As e-mail addresses are invariably instantly forgettable it makes sense to keep a record of them in an electronic address book. Addresses in this book can be 'pasted' into the *To*, *cc* and *Bcc* boxes.
Attachments	In addition to any text message you compose you can also attach other files to your e-mail. These may include documents you have created using a word processing package, spreadsheets, or images.
Send & Receive	Most e-mail programs allow you to compose your message offline – when you are not connected to the Internet. Messages sent whilst offline are stored in an Outbox. When you connect to the Internet you use the *Send and Receive* option to send any mail in your outbox and collect any mail that has been sent to you.

Attachments

In addition to being able to communicate with friends and colleagues through-out the world, e-mail also supports the use of attachments. As the name implies, an attachment is a digital file you attach to the e-mail. This may take the form of a word-processed document, an image or even a video clip. Without attachments e-mail would be limited to text messages.

Note, however, that attached files are typically large (in terms of file size) and consequently take longer to send and receive than simple text files. Moreover, the recipient of the e-mail will only be able to open the attachment if they have the appropriate piece of software. For example, if you attach a Microsoft Word file to an e-mail, the recipient will need a copy of this software or at least some other word-processing software that can read Word files.

Attachments – because they are binary files rather than simple text files – can also carry computer viruses. Consequently, before opening any attachment it is good practice to use a virus checker (see below).

Secure mail – encryption and digital signatures

Despite the many advantages e-mail offers, security is not one of its strengths. E-mails are akin to postcards inasmuch as the contents are not protected by a sealed envelope. However, whereas a postman or sorting clerk will tire long before they read anything to their advantage, a computer 'sniffer' programme, looking for trigger terms such as a credit card number or bank details, never will. Consequently, if you are going to use e-mail to send sensitive or confi-dential data some form of security is highly recommended. E-mails can be made secure through the use of encryption or digital signatures.

Encryption

With encryption the message you send is translated into a series of numbers and letters that can only be rendered meaningful if you have the encryption key.

The most popular form of encryption takes the form of public and private keys. Here, a piece of software is used to generate two alphanumeric keys. The private key is held on the user's computer and is never disclosed to anyone, whilst the public key is made available to everyone. Anyone can use this public key to send an encrypted message to this person, but only the intended recipient, who has the second part of the key, can decrypt the message.

If you are interested in using this type of encryption, an excellent piece of software, known as Pretty Good Privacy, can be downloaded free of charge from: <http://www.pgpi.com>.

Digital signatures

Digital signatures (known also as IDs and certificates) allow you to prove your identity in electronic transactions. In addition to having a public and private encryption keys, you also attach a digital signature to the e-mail that independently proves to the recipient that you are who you say you are, and that the message has neither been forged nor tampered with.

Digital IDs are issued by independent certifying authorities who verify your identity before issuing an ID. The leading certifying authorities are VeriSign <http://digitalid.verisign.com/> and British Telecom <http://www.trustwise.com/>. Both companies offer a free 60-day trial. If you wish to continue using your ID, the annual subscription fee is around £7.50.

Conventions and Netiquette

Unlike the telephone where your tone of voice adds meaning, or in a letter where a scented envelope would speak volumes, e-mail users can only determine meaning through the typed word. In an attempt to minimise the chance of being misunderstood various keyboard-codes have been devised. For example, to indicate that your comment is meant to be taken in jest the ;-) code is used. [If you tip your head through 90° you should get the idea of someone winking at you.] For more examples of these keyboard codes see: <http://www.pop.at/smileys/>.

Internet etiquette (netiquette) also dictates that e-mail messages should conform to the following rules:

- E-mails should be composed using lower case letters – If you use UPPER CASE IT LOOKS LIKE YOU ARE SHOUTING.
- E-mail signatures – a piece of text appended to each mail, that typically contains your name and contact details – should be no more than three lines long.
- Unless an attachment is going to significantly enhance the mail – do not use them.

Viruses

The final thing to consider when discussing e-mail is the potential threat of picking up a computer virus. A virus is a piece of software that has been written to secretly enter your computer system and 'infect' your files. Some viruses are benign and will not harm your computer, while others are destructive and can damage or destroy your data. Anyone doubting the power of computer viruses to cause widespread damage had a rude awakening with the distribution of the 'Love Bug' and 'Killer Resume' viruses. Both these viruses had the ability to damage computer programs, steal passwords, rename files and even redirect Web browsers – features millions of computer users all around the world became all too aware of. In financial terms the damage caused by the 'Love Bug' virus alone has been estimated to be in the region of $10 billion.

The distribution medium for both these viruses was e-mail. The beauty of e-mail, in the eyes of the people who author these viruses, is the ease by which the virus can be spread. As soon as anyone receives an 'infected' e-mail, all new mail that is sent from that computer carries the virus. This way the virus can continue to replicate itself.

To ensure that your computer does not become infected with a virus you need to install some anti-virus software. There are a number of suitable products on the market, many of which can be found at <http://dmoz.org/Computers/Security/Anti_Virus/Products/>. Once installed you need to subscribe to an update service to ensure that your system remains protected at all times.

Conclusion

Once you have set up and experimented with your Web browser and e-mail programs the potential of the Internet begins to become apparent. To help you exploit this potential we must now look beyond the basics and consider how we can search the Internet and find health information that is both timely and relevant.

Searching for information

Overview

The next three chapters focus on how you can search the Internet to find health information specific to your needs. With current estimates suggesting that there are in excess of 7 million Web sites and more than 2 billion Web pages, effective search tools and strategies are required if you are going to be successful in finding information that is accurate, timely, and appropriate to your requirements.

Chapter 4 looks at the different types of Internet search tools – search engines, Web directories, and evaluated gateways – and provides examples and analysis of how these can be used most effectively. Chapter 5 takes the concept of searching a stage further and looks at the key medical databases that can now be accessed via the Web. Particular attention is paid to providing a tutorial-like guide to searching MEDLINE, Cochrane Database of Systematic Reviews and the Complementary and Alternative Medicine Citation Index.

The Internet, however, is more than just a one-way channel of information. Through the use of Internet discussion lists and newsgroups, health consumers can share experiences and seek advice from people throughout the world who share a common interest. Chapter 6 introduces these services and provides tips and advice on how you can find discussion forums relevant to your interests.

CHAPTER 4

Searching the Web

Introduction

Searching for information on the Web is both deceptively easy and frustratingly difficult. Both Netscape Navigator and Internet Explorer have 'Search' buttons on their toolbars. When you click on this button you are automatically directed to a Web site where you can key-in your search terms to identify Web pages that contain information relevant to your search topic. Perhaps an even easier way of searching is simply to enter your search terms into the address bar on your browser. Once you hit the 'Enter' key you are again linked to the Microsoft or the Netscape search engine, where pages relevant to your search are displayed.

Though this method of searching is easy, the pages identified may not always be terribly useful or relevant. A search for information about migraine, for example, identified some 283,000 pages. And, though some of the pages identified were highly relevant – the Web sites of the Migraine Trust <http://www.migrainetrust.org/> and the *Bandolier* Migraine site <http://www.jr2.ox.ac.uk/Bandolier/booth/booths/migraine.html> are two such examples – there were others that were totally irrelevant. Anyone hoping to glean anything useful about this condition from sites such as the Migraine Boy – a comic strip character <http://www.slavelabor.com/migraineboypr.html> – and the Dark Planet Fiction site <http://www.sfsite.com/darkplanet/fiction/migraine.html> will be sadly disappointed.

The aim of this chapter is to provide you with the necessary skills to search the Internet effectively. To achieve this we will describe the different search tools currently available, highlight the relative strengths and weaknesses of each, and provide some tips to help ensure that whatever health topic you are researching on the Web you will find relevant and timely information.

Search tools

In December 1993 an e-mail message sent to the newsgroup <news://comp.infosystems.www> included a list of all the Web sites that were available on the Internet: the list detailed just 623 sites. Less than seven years later, the number of Web sites is estimated to exceed 7 million, whilst the number of pages on the Web was believed to be in excess of 2 billion. How many of these 7 million sites are relevant to health is difficult to say, but various surveys have indicated that well over 100,000 Web sites are exclusively dedicated to issues related to health.

With so much information available the practice of sending lists of Web sites to relevant newsgroups is now somewhat futile. Fortunately, various tools have been developed to help people navigate through this mass of data and discover information relevant to their interests.

In essence searching the Web requires the use of one or more of the following tools:

- Web search engines
- Web directories
- Evaluated subject gateways

Each method will identify different resources and which method you use will depend on what you are looking for and your own personal preferences. In this chapter we will discuss the key features of these tools, highlighting in particular how each method can be used to find health information on the Internet.

Search engines

Data from sources such as MediaMetrix <http://www.mediametrix.com/> show that Web search engines are – in terms of the traffic they receive – the most popular sites on the Internet. This is not surprising: at some point every Internet user wants to find information on the Web and search engines are the easiest way of achieving this.

To find information using a search engine you simply key-in your subject in the 'Search Box' at your preferred search site and press the 'Enter' key. Within a matter of seconds a list of Web sites is displayed that contain information relevant to your search topic. Figure 4.1 shows a search site (Google) and the results produced by a search for information on 'asthma'.

Search engines have been made possible by the development of computer programs knows as robots. Robot programs trawl the Internet in search of Web pages, images, videos etc. When a robot program finds a Web resource it takes a copy of all the words and images that are on that page and adds them to its database. As most Web pages have links to other pages the robot can follow those links and retrieve yet more pages. This process continues indefinitely. Thus, when you run a search, the search engine interrogates this database of Web pages.

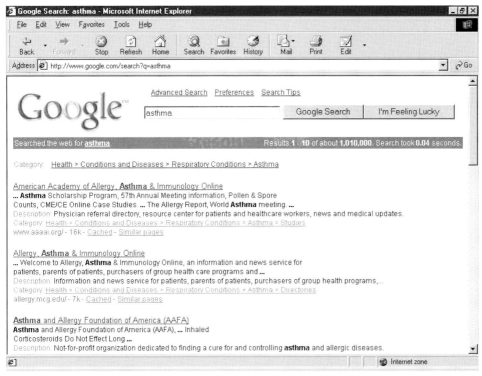

Fig. 4.1   Results page from Google

At present there are around a dozen or so popular search tools and all have their own strengths and weaknesses. Some are better at finding images, whilst others support more advanced search features that allow you to define your search more precisely.

Planning your search

For Internet searching to be effective – namely to find a small number of highly appropriate resources – some planning is required. Box 4.1 provides a number of tips to help you plan your search.

Whichever search engine you use it is important to remember that each one will produce different results (Box 4.2). Crucially, none of them indexes every page on the Web. Indeed, research undertaken by Inktomi and NEC Research Institute shows even the biggest search engine (Google) indexes little more than 50% of the Web.

Detailed below is a practical, quick reference guide to three of the best search engines currently available.

Box 4.1   Search tips

To help make your searching more effective consider the following:

- **Clarify your search**

  If you are simply looking for information on a single concept – migraine, asthma etc – then you have little choice other than to undertake a very simple single-word search. If, however, you are more interested in say the use of acupuncture in managing migraine or the relationship between air pollution and asthma, then adding these terms to your search query will help identify the more relevant sites.

- **Use Boolean logic**

  Once your search terms have been defined use the Boolean operators (Table 4.1) to refine or expand any search as required.

- **Be aware of synonyms**

  When using a search engine be alert to the need to consider using synonyms. For example, pages that provide information about breast cancer may use alternative terms such as 'breast neoplasms' or 'breast tumours'. If you wanted to find all pages relevant to this condition you would need to use all the synonyms in your search.

- **Be alert to variants in spelling**

  Similarly, be alert to variants in the way some terms are spelt. Continuing with the example cited above you would need to search for both 'brain tumour' and 'brain tumor' if your search was to identify all relevant pages.

  When searching for health information it is very important that you use the correct spelling. Hy**per**thyroidism and hy**po**thyroidism, for example, are two quite separate medical conditions. Spellings and definitions can be verified via the excellent online medical dictionary at: <http://medlineplus.adam.com>.

- **Think laterally**

  When trying to find the answer to a specific question try to think *where* the answer may have been published – rather than just keying in your question. For example, if you were trying to identify official statistics about the incidence of BSE/CJD in the United Kingdom the Department of Health would be a likely publisher of this type of data. Use Google to identify the Web address of this site.

Box 4.1   **Search tips** *(Continued)*

- **Use advanced search features**

  Most search engines offer two interfaces – one for simple searching and one for more complex searching. The 'Advanced' or 'Power' search interface will allow you to construct more complex searches – taking advantage of facilities such as proximity searching where you can specify that the terms you are looking for must appear within *x* number of words of each other, or in the same sentence.

Box 4.2   **Why different search engines produce different results**

A search undertaken on one search engine and then repeated on another will yield different results. Why?

- Different search engines may index different parts of the Internet. Remember that none of them indexes all the pages on the Web.
- Some search engines will try and gather everything they find at a Web site, whilst others will collect just a sample of Web pages.
- Some engines can successfully navigate (and thus index) image maps and Java-enabled pages – whilst others can not.
- All search engines weight the results in a slightly different way, which, if nothing else, gives the appearance of producing a different results-set. Google's ranking is partly based on the number of links to any site from any other site, whilst AltaVista uses a more usual ranking algorithm, based on the frequency of the terms searched for.

Google

<http://www.google.com>

Though a relative newcomer, Google has rapidly become one of the most highly respected search engines. With a reported index comprising of 560 million pages (plus links to a further 600 million pages) Google is the biggest Web search engine.

Searching with Google

To find relevant Web sites using Google you simply enter terms in the query box and press the *Google Search* button. The interface is clear, uncluttered and advertising-free. Once a search has been executed – which is surprisingly quick given the size of the index it has to search – you are told how many Web pages contain information relevant to the query, along with a list of these pages (Fig. 4.1).

What really differentiates Google from the other search sites, however, is the way it ranks the results. In addition to using standard text-matching algorithms – where ranking is determined by the frequency with which your search term appears – Google also employs a technique known as PageRank, which it defines in the following way:

> *PageRank relies on the uniquely democratic nature of the Web by using its vast link structure as an indicator of an individual page's value. In essence, Google interprets a link from page A to page B as a vote, by page A, for page B. But, Google looks at more than the sheer volume of votes, or links a page receives; it also analyses the page that casts the vote. Votes cast by pages that are themselves 'important' weigh more heavily and help to make other pages 'important'.*

A search using Google for Web sites that discuss asthma, for example, demonstrates the power of this ranking technology. Though such a simple search generated many hits – more than one million Web pages have information on this topic – at the top of this list were the Web sites of the American Lung Association <http://www.lungusa.org/asthma>, the American Academy of Allergy, Asthma and Immunology <http://www.aaaao.org> and the JAMA Asthma Information Center <http://www.ama-assn.org/special/asthma/asthma.htm>. All three sites are highly regarded and anyone looking for an authoritative overview of the disease will find these sites particularly useful.

Google's page ranking algorithm also makes it a particularly powerful tool when you are trying to find the home page of any known organisation.

The team behind Google are so confident that their search technology will identify the best site first that they invite users to select the 'I'm feeling lucky' button. On selecting this, users bypass the traditional search results page and instead are taken directly to the site Google ranks as being the most relevant to that search. In the asthma example cited above, selecting the 'I'm feeling lucky option' would have automatically redirected your browser to the Web site of the American Academy of Allergy, Asthma and Immunology.

Google also has an advanced search page <http://www.google.com/advanced_search> that supports a number of useful options including the facility to limit material to a particular language, and the opportunity to include (or exclude) pages from a defined domain. This latter option is very

Table 4.1   Boolean operators

Boolean operator	Syntax – with example	Consequence
AND	Migraine **AND** acupuncture	This search will only identify those Web pages where **both** terms are present.
		AND is used to refine a search.
OR	Migraine **OR** acupuncture	This search will identify any Web page where **either** term is present.
		OR is used to broaden a search.
NOT	Migraine **NOT** acupuncture	This search will identify all Web pages that contain the word migraine with the exception of those pages that also discuss acupuncture.
		NOT is used when you want to specifically **exclude** a particular concept.

useful if, for example, you want to restrict a search to pages that are in the '.uk' domain.

Anyone thinking that Google will address their entire search needs will, however, be disappointed to learn that key Boolean search operators (Table 4.1) are not supported. (Boolean search operators – AND, OR and NOT – allow you to construct more complex searches by combining or excluding specific concepts.)

By default Google uses the AND operator, and consequently only retrieves pages where all the terms are present. Google will not find those Web sites where *either* concept is discussed. This is a serious flaw when looking for health information as the same concept may be expressed in many different ways. 'Postnatal depression', 'postpartum depression' and 'baby blues' are all one and the same. Only by using the OR operator – which is not supported by Google – can you hope to perform an exhaustive search. Consequently, for more complex searches we must turn to other search engines, such as Northern Light and AltaVista.

Northern light

<http://www.northernlight.com>

Though its index of 265 million Web pages makes it smaller than Google, Northern Light has a sizeable collection of unique material, derived from a compilation of more than 7000 full-text magazines and newspapers. The Northern Light search engine can also undertake highly complex searches and, when necessary, these can be saved and automatically re-executed every time the database is updated.

Searching with Northern Light

When you search the Northern Light database both the Internet and the special collections database are searched. The special collections comprise full-text articles that are not readily available elsewhere on the Internet. Moreover, as this collection indexes a considerable number of medical titles – including the *British Medical Journal* and *The Lancet* – this can be a particularly valuable resource for those seeking authoritative health information. Articles indexed in the special collections attract a viewing fee, which typically costs between $1.00 and $4.00. Payment is made online via a secure, encrypted link.

The ability to undertake complex searching is another key feature of the Northern Light search engine. Via a simple to use 'Power Search' interface

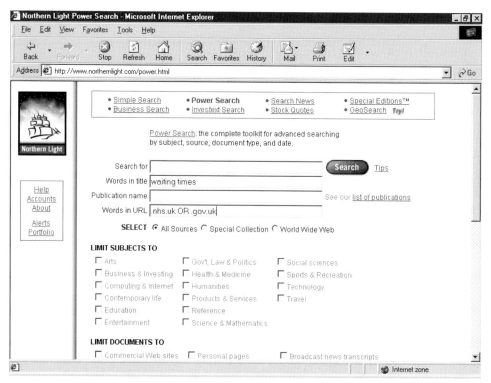

Fig. 4.2   Devising a complex search at Northern Light

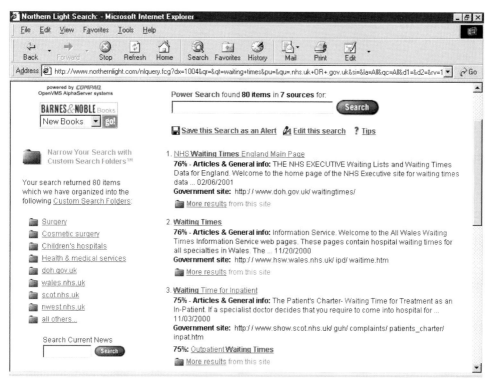

Fig. 4.3   Custom folders at Northern Light

<http://www.northernlight.com/power.html> it is possible to undertake a highly focused search that identifies a small number of relevant sites. For example, if you were trying to find data on waiting times, a search could be constructed that only finds those sites where the word 'waiting' appears in the title of the page and where the domain is either 'nhs.uk' or 'gov.uk' (Fig. 4.2).

Another unique aspect of the Northern Light database is the way search results are sorted into discrete 'custom folders' (Fig. 4.3). These folders group like data together based on the subject, source of the information (government, education, commercial etc) and language. Via a single mouse-click you can elect to view, say, pages that reside with the '.gov' (government) domain and ignore the personal home pages where the information tends to be more anecdotal and less credible.

Northern Light also has a 'Search Alert' service which can be used to identify new articles and Web sites that are of interest. To take advantage of this service you simply define a search and then save it as an 'Alert'. When the Northern Light database finds new Web pages (or articles in the special collection) that match your search query you are sent an e-mail informing you of this new information. No charges are levied to use this service.

AltaVista

<http://www.altavista.com>

For a number of years AltaVista was the search engine of choice. However, the emergence of new services like Google and Northern Light, coupled with the fact that AltaVista introduced an incredibly busy and advertising-heavy interface, has led to a decline in the popularity of this search engine. That said, AltaVista still has some unique search features that users searching for health information need to be aware of.

Searching with AltaVista

One of the strong features of the AltaVista search engine is the ability to be able to search the Web by media type. This is particularly useful if you are trying to identify whether there are any video or sound clips on the Web relevant to your chosen subject. Using this feature, and searching for videos related to 'heart surgery', we were directed to a number of clips including 'Heart surgery: an inside look', produced by NBC <http://www.msnbc.com> and 'Into the heart: a medical odyssey' <http://projo.com/special/heart/av.htm>. At the latter site there was a series of nine videos of pioneering surgeon Walt Lillehei describing and demonstrating how open heart surgery went from fantasy to medical reality. As Internet videos are presented in various formats (MPEG, Quicktime, Real Player etc) AltaVista allows you to limit the results of any search to those formats that you can view on your computer. [See Chapter 3, Table 3.1 for information on where these video players can be downloaded from.]

AltaVista also offers an 'Advanced' search interface. Using this it is possible to execute highly complex searches that use features such as nesting – where you can specify the order in which a search is executed – and the NEAR operator. NEAR is a useful weapon in the expert searcher's armoury as it allows you to find Web pages where the terms you are searching for are not necessarily adjacent to each other. For example, if you were interested in finding pages that discussed the role of surgery in the management of breast cancer then the search *'breast cancer' NEAR surgery* would identify relevant sites. More importantly, this search would *exclude* any pages where both concepts were discussed but were unrelated in the sense that the concepts were not discussed near one another. AltaVista defines NEAR as words that appear within 10 words of each other.

Table 4.2 provides a summary of the advanced search syntax used by AltaVista.

Table 4.2   AltaVista: advanced search syntax

Search	Syntax	Example	Result
Phrase searching	Enclose terms in double quotes – " "	"hormone replacement therapy"	Finds pages where this phrase occurs.
Combining terms – both have to be present	Use the **AND** operator	osteoporosis **AND** "hormone replacement therapy"	Only find pages where **both** concepts are discussed.
Either terms must be present	Use the **OR** operator	hrt **OR** "hormone replacement therapy"	Finds pages where **either** term is present.
Excluding terms	Use the **AND NOT** operator	osteoporosis **AND NOT** hrt	Finds only those pages that contain the term osteoporosis and **do not** contain the term hrt.
Terms must appear within 10 words of each other	Use the **NEAR** operator	osteoporosis **NEAR** hrt	The terms osteoporosis and hrt must occur within 10 words of each other.
Specifying the order a search should be executed	Use ( )	osteoporosis **NEAR** (hrt **OR** "hormone replacement therapy")	The search in brackets ( ) is executed first – and then if *either* word appears within 10 words of osteoporosis the page is retrieved.
Word stemming	Use the * symbol	"hormone replacement therap*"	Will find either therapy or therap**ies**.

Search engines – summary

Each of the search engines discussed here has its own strengths and weaknesses, which are summarised in Table 4.3. There are of course other Internet search engines available and a list of these (along with their key features) can be found at Danny Sullivan's excellent SearchEngine Watch site <http://www.searchenginewatch.com>.

Table 4.3   Search engine summary: quick reference guide

Service	Address	Strengths	Weaknesses
Google	<http://www.google.com>	• Largest index to the Web currently available • Best search tool for identifying home pages • Powerful page-ranking algorithm	• Difficult to perform complex Boolean searches
Northern Light	<http://www.northernlight.com>	• Unique collection of full-text magazines and newspapers • Complex searches can be constructed via simple pull-down menus • Results sorted into discrete subject-based folders • Alerting service available	• Relatively small database
AltaVista	<http://www.altavista.com>	• Option to search the Web by media type • Powerful advanced search options	• Cluttered and advertising-heavy interface

Web directories

The second approach to finding information on the Internet is to search (or browse) through one of the many Web directories that are now online. These directories attempt to classify Web resources into meaningful subject groupings. Thus, to find Web sites relating to say, alternative medicine, one simply accesses the alternative medicine catalogue, where material on this subject has been collected. Typically, Web directories are hierarchical in nature – a feature that allows you to 'drill down' to more specific subjects. Figure 4.4 shows how this hierarchy works in the area of health information.

One of the great strengths directory services have over automated, computer-compiled Web search engines is that they are created by people. A simple search for the term 'stroke' at Google, AltaVista etc will identify pages that discuss how you can become a better swimmer, or improve the

📁 Arts
📁 Business
📁 **Health**

    📁 Alternative Medicine
    📁 **Conditions and Diseases**

        📁 Allergies
        📁 Blood Disorders
        📁 **Cancer**

            📁 AIDS Related
            📁 Brain and CNS
            📁 **Breast**

                📁 Awareness
                📁 Breast Cancer Centers
                📁 **Treatment**

                    📁 Innovations in Breast care
                    📁 Mayo Clinic Cancer Resource Center

At each level in the hierarchy you can find sites that have information on that topic – or you can continue to drill down until you find a more specific term. In this example, the hierarchy was pursued through to those sites that specifically focused on the treatment of breast cancer.

Fig. 4.4 – Web directory – hierarchy of information

performance of your two-stroke motorcycle. Search engines are not smart, and cannot differentiate between different uses of the same words.

Web directories also allow you to identify Internet resources from a broad subject base, negating the need to search for highly specific terms. This can be a particularly useful feature if you are new to a subject and unsure of the best or most appropriate terminology. Moreover, the browseable nature of Web directories can alert to other broader, narrower and related terms, which may help you to define your subject search further.

When looking for health information two of the best subject directories are the Open Directory Project and the Karolinska Institute.

Open Directory Project

<http://dmoz.org>

The goal of the Open Directory Project (ODP) is to produce the most comprehensive directory of the Web. Unlike other directory services – such as Yahoo! <http://www.yahoo.com> the ODP relies exclusively on a vast army of volunteers. These volunteers, who have an interest in or knowledge of a specific subject, identify useful Web sites for the benefit of non-experts. Each subject category can have multiple editors – a factor that helps ensure that no one individual uses this directory to exclusively promote their own site or beliefs. At the time of writing, the ODP had some 30,000 editors who had indexed more than two million sites in 333,000 subject categories.

The easiest way to use this service is to search the entire directory. For example, a search for 'childbirth' will lead you to resources in various parts of the subject hierarchy such as:

- 'Health: Reproductive Health: Pregnancy and Birth: Childbirth',
- 'Health: Reproductive Health: Clinics and Services: Childbirth',
- 'Shopping: Health and Beauty: Reproduction and Sexuality: Pregnancy and Birth'.

Navigate to the first section identified and you are directed to around 210 sites that discuss all aspects of childbirth. If, however, childbirth is too broad a concept, you can select a narrower subject heading such as 'Caesarean and VBAC' (vaginal birth after Caesarean section) or 'Home Birth'. [As the ODP always displays the subject heading in relation to its position in the hierarchy, you can always move back up the hierarchy if you feel that the subject you have selected is too specific.]

At each subject-level a list of relevant Web sites is provided, and to help you determine which is the most appropriate to your information needs a brief one-line description is given (Fig. 4.5).

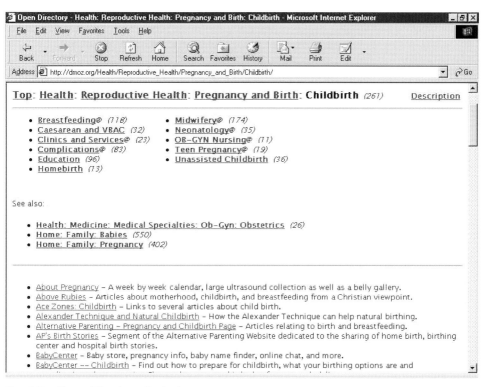

Fig. 4.5   Open Directory Project

Karolinska Institute

<http://www.mic.ki.se/Other.html>

Another useful Web directory has been compiled by staff from the Karolinska Institute in Sweden. Unlike the Open Directory Project, however, the Karolinska directory *only* contains links to biomedical Internet resources.

From the home page you can browse the resources from a broad subject perspective such as 'Ethics in Medicine and Science', and 'Diseases and Disorders and related Topics'. On following this latter link, all resources are then subject-classified using the MeSH [Medical Subject Headings] thesaurus developed by the US National Library of Medicine. This thesaurus, used to index articles in MEDLINE (see Chapter 5), is probably the best available tool for indexing medical resources. The MeSH thesaurus is arranged hierarchically. Osteoporosis, for example, is a narrower term within the joint-diseases hierarchy. In addition, because it uses a controlled vocabulary, MeSH groups like resources together. For example, the term 'heart attack' is mapped to the

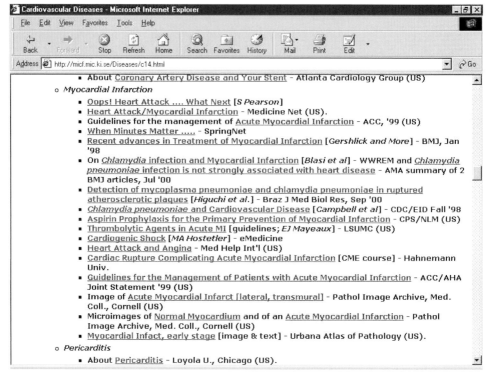

Fig. 4.6 Karolinska directory – Myocardial infarction section

preferred term 'myocardial infarction'. The advantage of this is that all resources appropriate to this condition are located together under one subject heading. Figure 4.6 shows the 'Cardiovascular Diseases' – 'Myocardial Infarction' section of this directory.

In addition to being able to identify relevant Internet resources using MeSH, you can also browse an alphabetical list of diseases <http://www.mic.ki.se/Diseases/alphalist.html> or do a keyword search against the Karolinska directory.

Though the Karolinska directory does not attempt to describe the resource it has indexed, it clearly shows the author/source of each resource. Using Figure 4.6 as an example, you can clearly see that some sites have been developed by individuals – the 'Opps – Heart Attack' site has been created by S. Pearson – whilst the 'Guidelines for the Management of Patients with Acute MI' have been developed by the American College of Cardiology and the American Heart Association. This information can be used to help determine which Internet sources are more authoritative. [The issue relating to the quality of health information on the Internet is discussed in Chapter 11.]

Other Web directories

If you wish to try out other directories consider Yahoo <http://uk.yahoo.com>, the first really popular Web directory, and still one of the most heavily trafficked sites on the Internet. A far less commercial alternative is the World Wide Web Virtual Library <http://vlib.org> and specifically the 'Medicine and Health' sections at <http://vlib.org/Medicine.html>.

Evaluated subject gateways

The third and final way to find health resources on the Internet is to use an evaluated subject gateway. In many ways these look and function much like the Web directories. The key difference, however, is that only those resources that meet defined (and published) quality criteria are included in the gateway directory.

Typically, evaluated subject gateway services will be created and maintained by a single organisation or by a group of dedicated individuals. Because each resource in the directory has to be identified and checked for quality, the number of Web sites indexed by these services is inevitably relatively small. Consequently, though these services will direct you to Internet sites of high quality, their coverage is somewhat limited.

Discussed below are three highly useful evaluated health information gateways.

MEDLINE*plus*

<http://www.medlineplus.gov>

Developed by the US National Library of Medicine, MEDLINE*plus* describes itself as 'a gold mine of up-to-date, quality health care information from the world's largest medical library'. Aimed specifically at health consumers – rather than professionals – MEDLINE*plus* provides access to extensive information about specific diseases and conditions. Additional information services include an online dictionary, a database of ongoing clinical trials and detailed drug information, derived from the US Pharmacopoeia. There is no advertising on this site, nor does MEDLINE*plus* endorse any company or product.

As with the other directory services, MEDLINE*plus* does not itself provide any information on any disease. It simply acts as a directory to high-quality Internet health resources.

Information on a specific subject can be identified by either searching the MEDLINE*plus* database, or by browsing the alphabetical list of subjects. Either

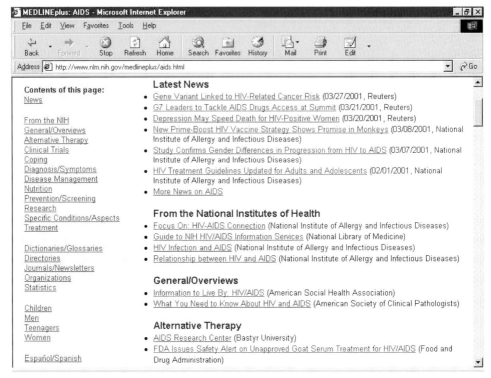

Fig. 4.7   MEDLINE*plus* – recommended AIDS resources

way, you will end up with an impressive list of highly useful Web sites. To help navigate each subject list, resources are sub-divided to enable you quickly to identify Web sites that focus on specific issues, such as treatment or diagnosis.

For example, on using the alphabetical list of diseases to navigate to Web resources that deal with 'AIDS', you are presented with a list of around 60 Web sites, categorised into 20 sub-topics. These range from general/overview-type sites (useful if you are new to this topic and want a quick overview), through to the more specific resources that discuss issues such as prevention and screening, alternative therapies, and ongoing research (Fig. 4.7).

All the Web resources in the MEDLINE*plus* directory meet strict, quality-assured guidelines. Central to these are the requirements that the source of the content is 'established, respected and dependable' and that information provided is 'appropriate to the audience level, well-organized and easy to use'. Emphasis is also given to those resources where the full-text content is available free of charge. Full details of the selection guidelines can be found at: <http://www.nlm.nih.gov/medlineplus/criteria.html>.

MEDLINE*plus* also provides users with a one-click approach to searching other key resources such as MEDLINE and the Clinical Trials database. MEDLINE (discussed more fully in Chapter 5) is the world's pre-eminent database for identifying current biomedical research. It is, however, a difficult database to search effectively, not least because of its size (over 11 million citations, dating back to 1966) and the fact that it uses a highly structured indexing vocabulary. Recognising these difficulties the team at MEDLINE*plus* have prepared a number of search strategies. All visitors need do is simply to select which search they would like to execute. Continuing with the example discussed above, MEDLINE searches have been prepared on topics such as 'AIDS prevention', 'AIDS diagnosis' and 'AIDS in infants and children'. On selecting any of these, a list of relevant citations – derived from articles published in peer-reviewed medical journals within the last six months – are delivered to your browser.

With regard to identifying ongoing clinical trials, again, prepared searches have been devised which can be used to interrogate the ClinicalTrials.gov <http://clinicaltrials.gov> database, developed by the National Institutes of Health (NIH).

MEDLINE*plus* is a truly remarkable resource and one that sets the standard to which other providers of health information need to aspire. The only problem with this service for UK health information seekers is that the material available at this site is aimed at US consumers. Though this does not matter in terms of finding information pertaining to the cause of a disease or what research is currently being undertaken, problems may arise when information about specific treatments is sought. A drug licensed in the US may not be available in the UK, or a clinical trial being conducted under the auspices of the NIH may not be open to UK patients. Equally, specific services such as those that help you identify the credentials of any US health professional <http://www.docboard.org> or what facilities are available at a specific hospital <http://www.ahd.com> are of little use to UK patients. It is time therefore to turn our attention to evaluated Web directories that are aimed specifically at a UK audience.

NHSDirect Online

<http://www.nhsdirect.nhs.uk>

Launched in December 1999 as part of the UK government's NHS Direct strategy, NHS Direct Online provides a gateway to high-quality patient information resources aimed at UK consumers.

The site has three main sections:

- Health features – a monthly magazine with hypertext links to related stories and sites
- Healthcare guide – an interactive guide to treating common symptoms at home

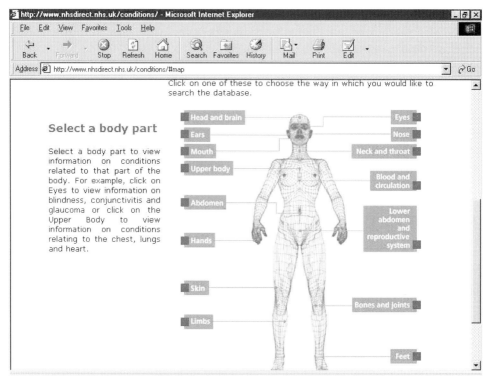

Fig. 4.8   Body map – NHSDirect Online

• Conditions and treatments – a database of information for patients on a variety of conditions.

By using the 'Conditions and Treatments' section, information on a specific disease can be accessed via an interactive body map, a keyword search, or by browsing an A-Z of topics. For example, using the body map (Fig. 4.8) and selecting, say, eyes, you are presented with a list of around 35 conditions that can affect this part of the body. This list includes the more obvious subjects like blindness and cataracts as well as highly specific conditions such as Treacher-Collins syndrome and Tuberous sclerosis.

On following a link to a specific disease the NHSDirect Online site directs you to relevant UK support groups and evaluated patient information leaflets and booklets. For a number of conditions, online audio and video clips are also available.

One of the problems with the NHSDirect site, however, is that many of the suggested information leaflets and booklets are not available online. The only way such information can be obtained is by writing to the organisation that has produced the material and requesting that they mail you a copy, for which there may be a charge. For an online information service this is somewhat disappointing and a factor that seriously undermines its usefulness.

Patient UK

<http://www.patient.co.uk>

The evaluated directory services discussed thus far are both government-sponsored sites. If you are looking for a more independent site the Patient UK service is highly recommended.

Developed by two UK GPs, Patient UK has been set up to provide patients with as much accurate and reliable information as they require. The directory, which links to hundreds of Web sites, can be both browsed and searched. When browsing, the user can select from broad subject categories, such as 'Staying Healthy' and 'Diseases and Illness', whilst a more focused user can make use of a cross-referenced alphabetical index.

Patient UK guides users in a stepwise fashion to sources of information of increasing complexity. Firstly, for each disease or health topic the user is directed to relevant support groups and appropriate online patient information leaflets. Secondly, any sources of drug information are then presented. Finally, the site provides the user with a number of links to more detailed information sources, such as original articles in professional journals and online guidelines. Users are also encouraged to look at a range of sites that focus on evidence-based medicine, and to search the MEDLINE database.

For example, on navigating to the 'Heart disease' section of the directory, links are provided to UK support groups such as the British Heart Foundation and the Family Heart Association, and to patient fact-files authored by various bodies such as the British Nutrition Foundation and the Cardiac Rehabilitation Research Unit. If more detailed information is sought, Patient UK then directs the user to a clinical guideline (Lipids and the Primary Prevention of Coronary Heart Disease) developed by the Scottish Intercollegiate Guidelines Network (SIGN) <http://www.show.scot.nhs.uk/sign/clinical.htm>, and to a collection of articles on heart disease, published in the *BMJ* <http://www.bmj.com/cgi/collection/ischaemic_heart_disease> (Fig. 4.9).

Though there is a degree of overlap with the NHSDirect Online service, the Patient UK directory directs the user to a number of unique sources of information that are highly credible. Consequently, if you wish to undertake a comprehensive search for high-quality UK Internet health sites you need to use both directories.

Other evaluated subject gateways

As discussed above, the coverage of each subject gateway is relatively small. For example, the MEDLINE*plus* directory identifies around 45 Internet resources for people seeking information about Alzheimer's disease. Notable

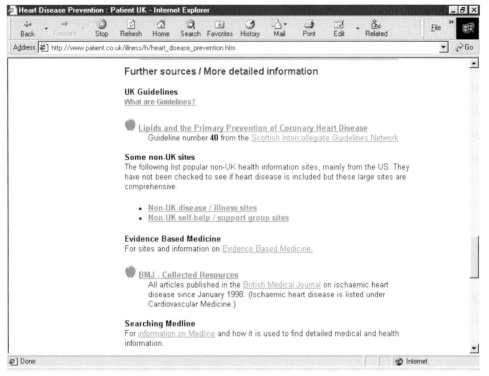

Fig. 4.9   Patient UK

absentees from this list include the respected 'Brain Briefings' from the Society for Neuroscience <http://www.sfn.org/briefings/> and Alzheimers.com <http://www.alzheimers.com>, a comprehensive online resource devoted to this subject.

Consequently, if you are looking for a comprehensive list of high-quality health Internet resources you will need to consider additional gateway sites. Others worthy of note include the Health on the Net Foundation <http://www.hon.ch>, OMNI <http://omni.ac.uk> and the MedWeb directory <http://www.medweb.emory.edu/MedWeb/> developed by Emory University.

Conclusion

This chapter has demonstrated the different methodologies you can use to find health information on the Internet. Which approach you employ will, in the main, be determined by what you are looking for and what you hope to find. When you seek just a few high-quality Internet resources the evaluated subject gateways should be your first choice. If a broader perspective is sought the more general Web directories are more appropriate. When highly specific

Table 4.4 Searching the Web: a summary

Search Tool	Examples	Use for ...
Search engines	Google, AltaVista & Northern Light	• Undertaking highly specific searches • Identifying large number of resources – irrespective of any quality filter
Web directories	Open Directory Project & Karolinska Institute Web Directory	• Identifying a broad spectrum of resources – though remember that these resources have not been subject to strict quality assurance selection guidelines
Evaluated subject gateways	MEDLINE*plus* & NHSDirect Online	• Identifying a small number of high-quality Internet resources

resources are required, a well-constructed query – using Boolean operators as appropriate – run against one of the Web search engines may prove to be highly effective. Table 4.4 provides a summary of the different search tools and highlights what type of question each tool is best suited to answering.

There is a vast amount of health information available on the Internet. Using the search tools, tips and techniques described here, relevant and appropriate information should never be more than a mouse-click away.

CHAPTER 5

Medical databases on the Internet

Introduction

The Internet has democratised health information. Sources such as clinical guidelines, drug compendiums and medical textbooks – which were previously only accessible to doctors and other health professionals – can now be accessed by anyone at the click of a button. Perhaps even more striking, however, is the fact that patients and their carers now enjoy equal (and free) access to a variety of research databases such as MEDLINE and the Cochrane Database of Systematic Reviews. Using these tools individuals can readily access current research and see what the state of knowledge is (referred to as the 'evidence-base') in any given topic.

Access to such tools significantly increases the sense of empowerment and in so doing makes the doctor–patient relationship more equal. For example, a pregnant woman who wanted to be able to raise questions in an informed way as to the best way to care for her unborn child and herself (is a home birth as safe as a hospital delivery? is one prenatal test safer than another? is zinc supplementation necessary? etc) would find the reviews produced by the Cochrane Pregnancy and Childbirth group most useful.

As stressed before, it is important that any information derived through such sources is shared and discussed with the appropriate healthcare team. Research that shows, for example, that a new drug has significant benefits may, if fact, be totally inappropriate in certain circumstances. The drug may only be suitable to a particular patient group or it may only be effective if the patient is not taking any other medication. Only the healthcare team have access to a patient's complete medical history and thus can make an informed judgement on how any piece of research can be applied to a specific patient.

With this proviso in mind, this chapter will discuss a number of freely available medical research databases and demonstrate how each can be searched to find timely and relevant information.

Search engines or medical databases?

Before we look in detail at a number of online medical databases it is important to clarify that the information contained within each database **cannot** be found through the use of the Internet search engines (Chapter 4).

Medical databases, like MEDLINE, form part of the 'invisible Web' – resources that can be accessed on the Web, but ones whose contents cannot be directly accessed by Internet search engines. Put another way, an Internet search engine will be able to find the MEDLINE home page, but would not be able to interrogate the MEDLINE database directly. Consequently, to search MEDLINE (and all the other databases discussed here) one must access the database home page and run the search from there.

Medical databases

There are many databases health professionals can turn to when trying to determine what research has been published on a given topic. A researcher considering the ethical implications of *in vitro* fertilisation (IVF) would find the BioethicsLine database a rich source of information. Equally, a physician with an interest in cancer would appreciate the wealth of information available through the CancerLit database.

Probably the two most useful medical research databases, however, are MEDLINE and the Cochrane Library of Systematic Reviews. In this chapter special attention will be given to these databases and, in recognition of the growing interest in complementary medicine, the Complementary and Alternative Medicine Citation Index will also be discussed. The chapter will conclude with a brief look at a number of the more subject-specific databases.

MEDLINE

<http://www.ncbi.nlm.nih.gov/PubMed>

MEDLINE, produced by US National Library of Medicine, is the world's premier biomedical database. Dating from 1966 (though the printed version, Index Medicus, dates from 1879) the MEDLINE database currently contains over 11 million bibliographic references and abstracts drawn from more than 4300 biomedical journals.

The database is primarily used to identify published research on a specific topic. Crucially, as MEDLINE only indexes articles that have been published in peer-reviewed journals – all articles have been independently reviewed and approved – the information is generally of high quality. [Inevitably, there will be *some* articles that had they been more rigorously reviewed may not have been published, and subsequently indexed by MEDLINE. As a rule of thumb, however, references from a MEDLINE search can be trusted.]

When searching MEDLINE it is important to remember that it is a bibliographic database. Though you will be able to identify key papers and read online abstracts, in the overwhelming majority of cases you will not be able to get to the full-text of an article. Recognising the limitation of this, the developers of MEDLINE have recently introduced a system whereby publishers can create hypertext links to full-text articles. At the present time, however, the number of publishers who allow their full-text journals to be freely accessible through MEDLINE is disappointingly small.

Searching MEDLINE

As with Internet search engines, searching MEDLINE is both deceptively easy and frustratingly difficult. Simply by entering any term or phrase into the MEDLINE search box you will identify relevant-sounding articles. A search for 'multiple sclerosis', for example, retrieves some 21,250 references on this topic. Some of these may be of interest to you, and some will not. Determining which is which from a list of this size, however, will depend upon one's luck and diligence, and since these may be in short supply, it makes more sense to devise more sophisticated searches that focus on a particular aspect of the disease. The following sections provide guidance on how such searches can be constructed.

Before constructing any MEDLINE search, however, check the MEDLINE*plus* site (discussed in Chapter 4) to determine whether a predefined search on the topic you wish to research has already been devised.

Basic searching

Though MEDLINE uses a highly structured vocabulary (see 'Advanced searching' below) it is nevertheless possible to search for articles using common terms and phrases. The search 'preventing flu', for example, identifies a number of potentially useful articles (Fig. 5.1), including one from a recent issue of the journal *JAMA* entitled 'Preventing influenza in healthy adults' and another from the *American Journal of Managed Care* with the title 'Advances in the prophylaxis and treatment of influenza illness'. In this example, the *JAMA* article was available in full-text free of charge, whilst the other reference was supported by a detailed online abstract (Fig. 5.2).

Though these articles would prove useful, a quick glance at the results-page (Fig. 5.1) shows that others would not. Unless you speak Hebrew, the first reference would be irrelevant, as would those that deal with flu as it pertains to specific conditions, such as asthma and cystic fibrosis.

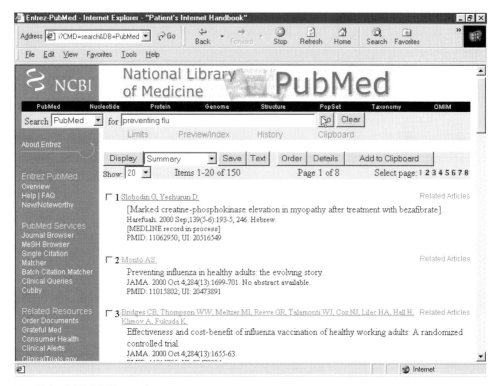

Fig. 5.1   MEDLINE search screen

Rather than having to sift though a list of irrelevant articles it makes more sense to refine a search though the use of the 'Limits' menu. On selecting this, search results can – amongst other things – be limited to articles that have been published in a specific language and within a defined time frame. In the example cited above, limiting this search to articles that were published in English, within the past two years, reduced the number of references to a more manageable 32. Box 5.1 provides a worked example of refining a search through the 'Limits' option.

Intermediate searching

The searching so far has been limited to a single concept. More often than not, however, MEDLINE is searched to find articles that discuss the relationship between multiple concepts. The link between asthma and air pollution or the possible causal relationship between leukaemia and high-frequency power lines are but two examples.

To undertake this more sophisticated type of searching you need to input

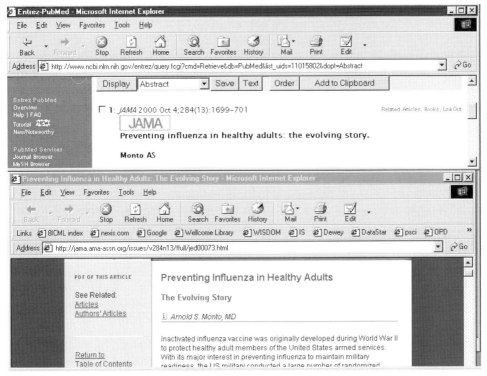

Fig. 5.2   MEDLINE citation with links to full-text articles

each concept, one at a time, and then combine them using the Boolean operators, as discussed in Chapter 4, Table 4.1.

Box 5.1 provides a stepwise example of how such a search can be constructed.

Advanced searching

All the articles in the MEDLINE database are indexed using MeSH (Medical Subject Headings). One of the advantages of using such a controlled vocabulary is that like-resources are grouped together, irrespective of the specific terms individual authors may have used in their work. For example, one author may use the term 'baldness' whilst another may use 'alopecia' to describe the same condition. MeSH overcomes the problem of synonyms by forcing indexers to use a set of preferred terms. As a consequence, MeSH searching is far more precise than simple free-text searching.

MeSH searching can be enhanced further through the use of appropriate subheadings – such as diagnosis, epidemiology, and therapy. A search that uses

Box 5.1   Intermediate MEDLINE searching

In this example, MEDLINE is used to find articles that discuss the relationship between asthma and air pollution. The search is then limited to articles published in English within the past two years, and where the focus of the study is children, aged 6–12.

1. Go to the MEDLINE database <http://www.ncbi.nlm.nih.gov/PubMed>

2. In the **Search** box, enter the term *asthma* – click the **Go** button

   A list of citations that contain the term 'asthma' are displayed – 20 references at a time.

3. Next, use the **Clear** button to empty the search box and then enter the phrase *air pollution* – click the **Go** button. Note: When inputting terms into the MEDLINE database do **NOT** put quotation marks around any term or phrase.

   Two separate sets of results have now been created. Set 1 contains articles about asthma, whilst Set 2 has articles on air pollution. These sets now need to be combined using the AND operator.

4. Click on the **History** button to see your search history.

   In this example you will see two sets – one for each subject we have searched for – along with the number of articles MEDLINE has retrieved.

5. Use the **Clear** button to empty the search box and enter the set numbers you want to combine. When combining search sets always prefix the set number with the # character. Boolean operators, AND, OR, and NOT **must** be entered in upper case.

   In this example we enter:

   #1 AND #2

   Press **Go**

   As this search produced over 3000 references, various limits can be applied to focus the search to the more pertinent articles.

6. Click on the **Limits** option (Fig. 5.3).

   From the subsequent menu, use the **Entrez Date** option to limit the results to articles published in the past two years. Use the **Language** option to restrict the articles to those that have been published in English. Use the **Age** option to limit the search to those articles that focus on children, age 6–12. Click **Go** to apply these limits.

Limiting the search in this manner reduced the number of retrieved references from 3019 to 167.

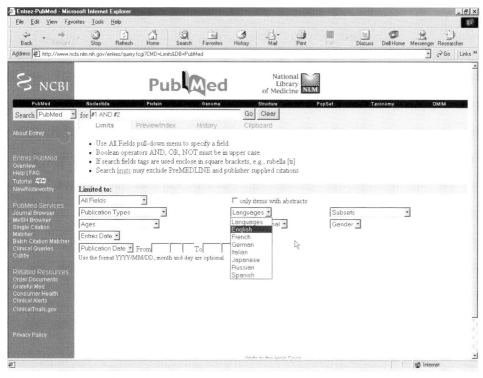

Fig. 5.3   MEDLINE limits menu

the subheading 'diagnosis' will *only* find those articles that discuss this specific concept. More wide-ranging articles, such as those that look at how a disease could be prevented or treated etc, would be discarded from the search results.

Box 5.2 details how an advanced search, that makes use of MeSH terms and subheadings, can be constructed.

Other searches

Limiting a search to full text articles
As discussed above, there are a (small) number of publishers who make the full-text of published articles accessible via MEDLINE. As yet, however, there is no 'limit' function within MEDLINE that allows a user to restrict a search to just those papers that are freely available on the Web. Recognising this, the developers of the Hardin Meta Directory of Internet Health Resources <http://www.lib.uiowa.edu/hardin/md/> have compiled a list of freely avail-able, full-text journals that are indexed by MEDLINE. On selecting this link

Box 5.2   Advanced MEDLINE searching

*In this example, MEDLINE is used to find articles on shingles –
particularly those that look at the epidemiology and the prevention
and control of this disease.*

1. Go to the MEDLINE database
   <http://www.ncbi.nlm.nih.gov/PubMed>

2. Using the MEDLINE toolbar (Fig. 5.1) click on the **MeSH browser**
   option (located under PubMed Services) and in the subsequent
   dialogue box enter the term *shingles* – click the '**Go**' button.

   On doing this MEDLINE reports the following: **shingles** *is not a
   MeSH term, but it is associated with the MeSH term* **Herpes Zoster**.
   *A definition of the term is also provided and on scrolling down this
   page you will see where Herpes Zoster fits into the MeSH hierarchy.*

3. Click on the **Detailed display** option.

   *The resulting display shows all the MeSH subheadings that can be
   applied to this term. These include 'complications', 'drug therapy',
   and 'radiotherapy'.*

4. Select the subheadings relevant to this search – **prevention and
   control** and **epidemiology**. This is achieved by clicking the check-box
   adjacent to each heading.

5. Because we are interested in articles that discuss either the
   epidemiology of shingles <u>or</u> the prevention and control of this viral
   disease, select the **OR** search operator and then click on the option
   to **Add** terms to search.

6. These terms are then pasted into the Search box. To run the search,
   click the **PubMed Search** button.

   *The search could be refined further by combining additional search
   terms and by introducing limits, as discussed in Box 5.1.*

What this search successfully highlights is the importance of using
MeSH terms if you want to undertake a comprehensive search. All
relevant articles – whether they contain the word 'shingles' or the
more technical term 'herpes zoster' – are successfully retrieved in
one search set.

<http://www.lib.uiowa.edu/hardin/md/ej.html> a MEDLINE search is executed which brings together, in one result set, all MEDLINE articles that are available in full-text. All you then have to do is to add the search term(s) you are interested in and combine both sets of results.

Finding papers by a known author
To find papers by a known author, enter the name in the format of *last name* plus *initials*. A search for kiley r, for example, would direct you to papers written by this author. It would, however, also find papers written by kiley ra, kiley rb etc. To disable this automatic truncation facility use double quotes around the author's name and specify the author search-field tag [au], as shown below:

"kiley r"[au]

Viewing and printing MEDLINE references
Once a search has been executed on MEDLINE the results are displayed in a summary format. Information provided here includes the author(s), title of the article and publication details. Box 5.3 shows how the display can be changed and relevant citations printed.

Box 5.3   **Viewing and printing MEDLINE references**

- To view online abstracts click on the pull-down menu adjacent to the 'Display' option, select **Abstract** and then click on the **Display** tab (Fig. 5.4)

  Though every citation displayed can be printed, it is probably more useful to scan each reference and select for printing just those which sound most useful.

- To select a citation, simply click the **check-box** – adjacent to each citation. Continue to do this – one page at a time – until all the references have been looked at.

- When you have finished, click on the box **Add to clipboard**. All the citations you have marked now appear in one new set – ready for you to print.

- To print the citations use the **Print** button, located on the browser's toolbar.

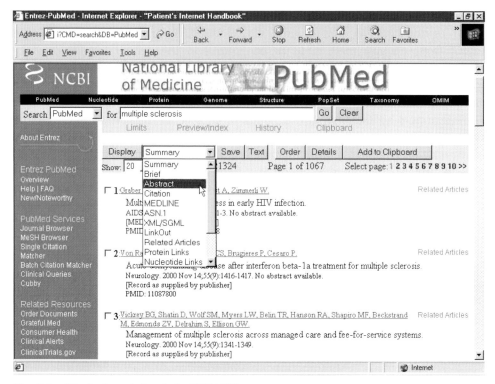

Fig. 5.4   Displaying abstracts in MEDLINE

Further help

For further information and help on how to search MEDLINE effectively see the MEDLINE Training manuals, written by staff of the National Library of Medicine. These can be accessed at: <http://www.nlm.nih.gov/pubs/web_based.html>. For a less in-depth analysis see the *PubMed: a cheat sheet* guide at: <http://www.nahec-wi.org/pubmedc.htm>.

Cochrane Database of Systematic Reviews

<http://www.update-software.com/cochrane/cochrane-frame.html>

The Cochrane Database contains a series of original reviews that attempt to determine whether treatments for specific and identified conditions are effective. Conclusions are reached by looking at *all* the research that has been published on a defined topic. Recognising that some pieces of research are more authoritative than others, the authors of the Cochrane Reviews focus on research that was conducted using the randomised controlled trials (RCTs) methodology. Studies conducted using RCTs are less prone to bias and produce more reliable conclusions.

Each review in the database is highly structured and provides the user with information on the study's objectives, the main results and the conclusions that can be drawn. Moreover, each review is clearly dated and, as new research becomes available, subject to change.

Although the complete, full-text version of this database is not freely available on the Internet, all the abstracts (which include the main results and conclusions) are accessible without charge.

The only major problem with this database is its size. At the time of writing the total number of reviews was around one thousand. And, though some groups such as the Pregnancy and Childbirth and the Neonatal groups have commissioned a significant number of reviews (167 and 96 respectively), other groups are not so well developed. The Heart Group for example has just four reviews, one more than that produced by the Hypertension Group. Inevitably, therefore, there will be occasions when the Cochrane Database is unable to help.

Searching the Cochrane Database

The easiest way to identify relevant, evidence-based reviews is to search the database. In contrast to the sophisticated way MEDLINE can be searched, however, this version of the Cochrane Database only supports simple free-text searching. Even more disappointing is the fact that Boolean searches are unsupported, thus rendering it impossible to construct a well-defined search strategy. For example, a search for reviews that discuss the effectiveness of acupuncture in helping someone to stop smoking identifies seven reviews. Though one of these was highly relevant ('Acupuncture for smoking cessation'), others were irrelevant, and were only identified because they contained one of the search terms.

A worked example of how the Cochrane Database can be searched is provided in Box 5.4.

Another way to identify relevant reviews is to browse the database, using the Cochrane Collaborative Review Group headings. There are around 50 of these groups, covering topics such as breast cancer, schizophrenia and epilepsy.

For example, on selecting the Peripheral Vascular Diseases Group the titles of some 17 reviews are displayed. Any relevant-sounding review can be selected and the full Cochrane abstract is displayed on the screen.

If you want access to the *full* Cochrane Database – which includes the full text of all topic reviews (not just the abstracts) and the Cochrane protocols – this is available as a subscription service (£120.00 per year). It should also be pointed out that the subscription version offers a far more sophisticated search

Box 5.4   Searching the Cochrane Database

For many years ginger has been promoted as a safe and effective way of preventing nausea, particularly in early pregnancy. In this example, the Cochrane Database is searched to see if there is any hard evidence to support this popular belief.

1. Go to the Cochrane Library <http://www.update-software.com/cochrane/cochrane-frame.html>

2. From this page follow the link to Cochrane Abstracts <http://www.update-software.com/abstracts/Default2.htm>

3. In the search box enter the single term **ginger**. Click on the **Search** button.

   This search identified just one review, entitled 'Interventions for nausea and vomiting in early pregnancy'. (Fig. 5.5)

   On selecting this review, the full abstract is displayed on the screen. Though a whole range of treatments for managing nausea in early pregnancy is discussed, specific reference is made to the use of ginger. In this case, the Cochrane reviewers conclude that 'ginger may be of benefit, but the evidence so far is weak'.

If you were interested in finding out what other reviews had been written that discuss the best ways of caring for pregnant women and their new-born babies, click on the Cochrane Abstracts link <http://www.update-software.com/abstracts/mainindex.htm> and navigate to those reviews conducted by the Cochrane Pregnancy and Childbirth Group.

If you need to see the full text of any Cochrane review – but do not want to commit yourself to an annual subscription – the online document delivery service may be of use. The fee and delivery schedule can be seen online at: <http://www.updateusa.com/Document_Delivery/Doc-Delivery.html>

interface that supports MeSH and Boolean searching. Further details of this service can be found at: <http://www.update-software.com/cochrane/orderform-cochrane.html>.

[*Note: As this book was going to press a consumer version of the Cochrane Database became available on the Internet. Here, short readable summaries of*

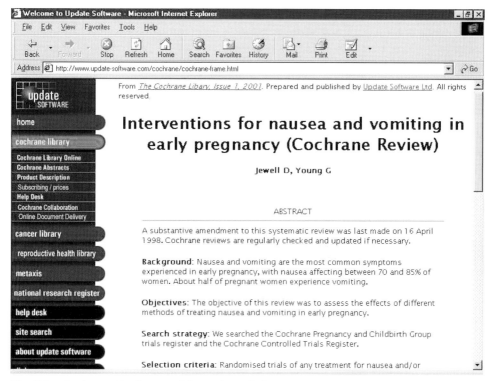

Fig. 5.5   Cochrane Review – evidence-based abstracts

the Cochrane Reviews are available. To access this resource point your browser at: <http://www.cochraneconsumer.com/>.]

Complementary and Alternative Medicine Citation Index (CCI)

<http://nccam.nih.gov/nccam/resources/cam-ci/>

Interest in complementary and alternative medicine (CAM) has never been greater. Indeed, it has been estimated that over 5 million UK citizens consulted a CAM practitioner in the past year. In an attempt to help consumers make more informed decisions about CAM the US National Center for Complementary and Alternative Medicine has developed the CAM Citation Index (CCI). CCI is a searchable database that consists of around 175,000 CAM-related bibliographic citations, dating from 1963 to the present.

Data in the CCI is derived predominantly from the MEDLINE database. Though this means that one could ignore the CCI database – all the data in CCI is duplicated in the parent database MEDLINE – the Citation Index offers any-one researching into CAM some unique search features. Prominent amongst these is the fact that the database can be searched by CAM system, or by CAM method. Such features are not supported by the MEDLINE database.

Searching the CCI database

Visitors to the CCI Web site are presented with two search options – basic and expert – and a browse facility. As its name implies, the expert search option facilitates the construction of more complex and refined searches, through the use of Boolean operators and field-specific searching. Box 5.5 shows a worked example of how the advanced search features were used to find a small number of highly relevant articles.

The developers of the CCI have also developed a highly effective browsing tool. Using this option one can select references that focus on a specific form of CAM, such as hypnotherapy or acupuncture, or those that pertain to a particular CAM system, such as Ayurvedic medicine, or homeopathic medicine. The database can also be browsed by disease.

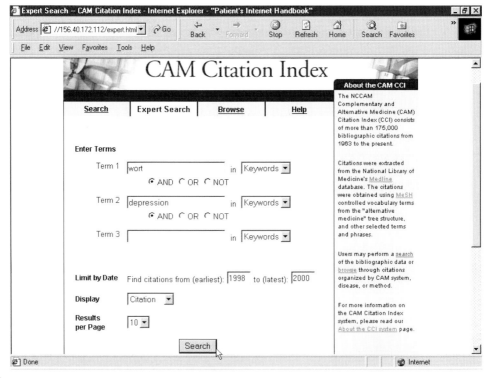

Fig. 5.6   Expert searching of the CAM CCI

Box 5.5   Searching the CAM Citation Index – expert mode

In this example the CAM Citation Index is searched to find articles that discuss the use of St John's Wort in managing depression, published in the past two years.

1. Go to the Cam Citation Index – Expert Search Page
   <http://156.40.172.112/expert.html>

2. Using the on-screen search form (Fig. 5.6), the term **wort** is entered into the Term 1 search box.

   *As at this stage you may wish to keep the search fairly broad, select the **ALL** option from the pull down menu. If this identifies too many hits, select Title or Abstract from the field-limiting menu to refine the search.*

3. In the Term 2 search box enter the term **depression**. Again, this search term is not limited to a particular field.

4. Check that the **AND** radio-type button is selected. Remember, in this example we were looking for articles that discuss both concepts.

5. Use the **Limit by Date** function to restrict the search to articles published in the past two years.

6. Click on the **Search**-button to run the search.

   In this example, some 21 references were found.

7. Scan through the results list, marking any (by use of the check-box facility) that sound interesting. Once you have been through the complete set of references the **Display** button can be used to see the selected citations in more detail.

The real strength of this browse facility, however, is that all these options can be combined. Figure 5.7 shows how the browsing option can be employed to identify research into the use of acupuncture in treating back pain. As this search produced over 160 citations, the browse facility was used further to restrict the search to articles published since 1995, and to those studies that were conducted using randomised-controlled trials. Introducing these limits reduced the number of references to just seven, including one from the *Archives of Internal Medicine* with the title 'Acupuncture for back pain: a meta-analysis of randomized controlled trials'.

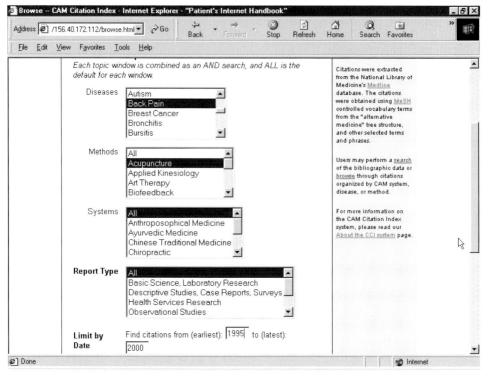

Fig. 5.7   Browsing the CAM CCI

Other subject-specific databases

In addition to the databases described here there are a number of other subject-specific databases, freely accessible via the Internet. Brief details of these are provided in Table 5.1.

Conclusion

The wealth of resources available via these online databases is staggering. The MEDLINE database alone indexes over 400,000 new articles every year. Being aware of these resources and, more importantly, developing the skills to interrogate them effectively, can significantly heighten the patient's sense of empowerment. Indeed, speaking at the launch of the free MEDLINE service in 1997, heart surgeon Michael de Bakey famously remarked that 'good informa-tion is the best medicine'. Using the resources highlighted here, everyone – patients, carers as well as health professionals – can now access this body of research to help make informed decisions about effective patient care.

Table 5.1   Subject-specific databases: a quick reference guide

Database: AIDSLINE
Address   <http://igm.nlm.nih.gov>
Size   200,000 citations
Coverage: 1980 to date
Analysis   This database provides access to research on AIDS and related topics. In
           addition to indexing journal articles, AIDSLINE also provides access to US
           government reports, conference papers and books.

Database: BIOETHICSLINE
Address   <http://igm.nlm.nih.gov>
Size   60,000 citations
Coverage: 1973 to date
Analysis   Produced by the Kennedy Institute of Ethics at Georgetown University,
           BIOETHICSLINE provides access to research that focuses on the ethical
           issues in healthcare and biomedical research. Topics covered include
           euthanasia, organ transplantation and abortion.

Database: CancerLit
Address   <http://cnetdb.nci.nih.gov/cancerlit.shtml>
Size   1.5 million citations
Coverage: 1960 to date
Analysis   Produced by the US National Cancer Institute's International Cancer
           Information Center, CANCERLIT contains references to the vast body of
           cancer literature published from the 1960s to the present. CANCERLIT is
           updated with more than 8000 records every month.

Database: Clinical Trials Database
Address   <http://www.clinicaltrials.gov>
Size   5000 clinical studies – primarily those sponsored by the US National
           Institutes of Health
Coverage: 1997 to date
Analysis   The Clinical Trials database aims to 'link patients to medical research'.
           Trials can be identified by searching the database or browsing by disease
           condition. Each trial in the database contains a description
           highlighting its purpose, what phase it has reached, and whether or not
           new recruits are still being accepted.

Database: National Research Register
Address   <http://www.update-software.com/National/nrr-frame.html>
Size   68,000 research projects
Coverage: 1998 to date
Analysis   The National Research Register is a database of ongoing and recently
           completed research projects funded by, or of interest to, the United
           Kingdom's National Health Service. In addition to the 68,000 research
           projects, the database can be used to identify clinical trials funded by the
           Medical Research Council and details on reviews in progress collected by
           the NHS Centre for Reviews and Dissemination.

CHAPTER 6

Discussion lists and newsgroups

Introduction

One of the undoubted strengths of the Internet is the ease with which we can communicate with friends and colleagues throughout the world. As discussed in Chapter 3, if you know someone's e-mail address you can be assured that the mail will reach that recipient, typically within a few minutes of being sent.

In addition to this one-to-one communication, the Internet also provides the opportunity to communicate on a one-to-many basis through the use of online discussion forums. Here, people with a common interest – such as a particular medical condition, a hobby, or a work-related topic – come together, via e-mail, to share experiences and seek advice.

For example, a patient with a prostate disease may wish to join the *Prostate Problems* discussion list <http://listserv.acor.org/archives/prostate.html>. This group, which has almost 1700 subscribers, 'welcomes all those with involvement or interest in prostate problems – patients, loved ones, health care professionals, and other concerned people interested in participating in an honest discussion of concerns, treatment options, and general information on prostate problems'. Issues raised in recent months included discussion of the efficacy of fish oil supplements, debate over the price of the drug Casodex, as well as a number of postings from people who have recently been diagnosed with prostate cancer and were looking for general information and support.

Indeed, the support element of these discussion forums is probably their greatest asset. Karen Parles, a librarian from New York who was diagnosed with lung cancer, spoke of the value of online discussion forums:

> *I found a great support group for lung cancer, the Lung-Onc mailing list. The other patients on the list answered my questions, suggested useful sites, and gave me a lot of invaluable support.*

On being told she would need a lung removed Karen again turned to the group:

Having a lung removed by an unproved procedure still seemed pretty frightening, so I shared my fears with my Lung-Onc friends. I heard right back from eight or ten others who'd had a pneumonectomy. They assured me that I could do it and encouraged me to give it a shot.

The group was a great source of advice for dealing with day to day problems during my recovery. Patients who've had chest surgery often have trouble sleeping because every possible position makes your ribs hurt. The folks on the list can tell you exactly what to do.

[For the full story, see the article by Tom Ferguson in the *BMJ*, 4 November 2000, available online at:
<http://www.bmj.com/cgi/content/full/321/7269/1129>.]

Through such discussion lists patients and their carers can get first-hand advice and support from fellow sufferers. And, though information found through such forums – especially if it pertains to particular therapeutic regimes – should be discussed with your doctor, the value of being able to share common experiences is widely recognised. Moreover, if you are caring for someone with a relatively rare condition the chances of you actually meeting anyone in a similar position is somewhat limited. In the online environment, however, you can interact with fellow carers, irrespective of their geographical location.

In this chapter we are going to look at the two forms of online discussion – discussion lists and newsgroups – and discuss how you can find online forums that pertain to your specific interests. In addition to this we will give some practical advice on how you join (and leave) discussion forums and discuss some of the issues you need to consider before you mail your first set of questions and comments.

Discussion lists

Discussion lists (also know as mailing lists) are subject-based discussion groups that are participated in and distributed by e-mail. Once you have joined a list – for example, the *Lung-Onc* list mentioned above – a copy of every message that is posted to this list is sent to your electronic mailbox. As a computer performs the task of copying and forwarding mail messages to every list member, the effort for the individual is the same as sending any other e-mail. No charges are levied to join any list.

Finding lists relevant to your interests

With recent estimates suggesting that the number of Internet discussion lists exceeds 90,000, the greatest problem any Internet user faces is identifying relevant lists. This problem is exacerbated by the fact that there is no single directory service that brings all these disparate lists into one searchable database.

With this proviso in mind, the Liszt Mailing List Directory <http://www.liszt.com/> is a useful starting point. Here, relevant discussion lists can be identified by keyword searching the database. For example, a search for Creutzfeldt–Jakob disease identifies one relevant list, *CJDVOICE*. In addition to this basic data the Liszt database also provides information on how to join the list, its purpose and whether there is a related Web site where further information can be found.

Another useful source is Yahoo! Groups <http://groups.yahoo.com>. Here discussion lists can be identified by keyword searching, or by browsing the Yahoo! Groups hierarchy.

If a search of these sources yields nothing, the best approach is to use one of the evaluated health gateways discussed in Chapter 4. Of particular note is the Emory MedWeb directory, <http://www.medweb.emory.edu/MedWeb/> where an A–Z list of health discussion forums has been compiled. To facilitate navigation of this resource, all the discussion lists have been subject-indexed and placed in a hierarchical directory (Fig. 6.1). On following the link to

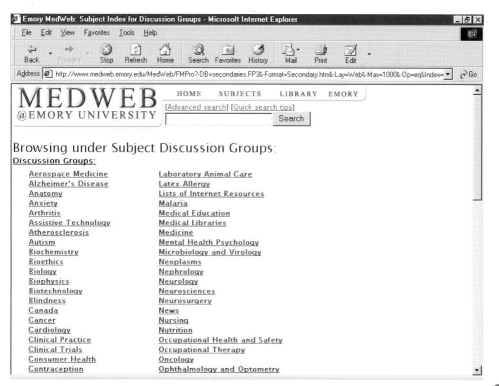

Fig. 6.1   Subject indexing for discussion lists – Emory MedWeb

Pregnancy, for example, you are directed to just two resources, each of which, however, provides details of numerous pregnancy-related discussion lists.

Section 5 of this book provides details of discussion lists for 100 common diseases and conditions.

Joining and contributing to a discussion list

Once you have identified a relevant discussion group the next step is to join the list so that messages sent to the list appear in your mailbox. Joining any list simply requires you to send an e-mail to the listserver that hosts the list,

Box 6.1   Joining the *Prostate Problems* discussion list

Note that this message is sent to the listserver.

To: listserv@listserv.acor.org

Subject: leave blank

Text: subscribe PROSTATE *firstname surname*

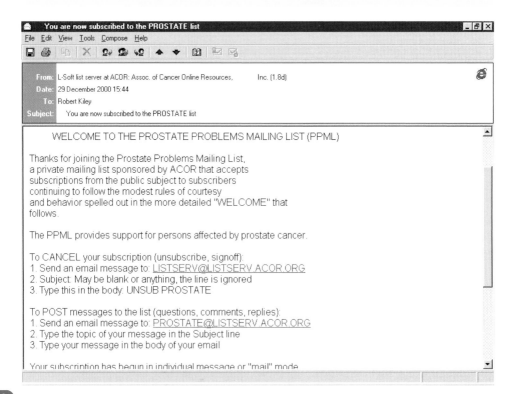

Fig. 6.2   Welcome message from the *Prostate* list

indicating which list you wish to subscribe to. Box 6.1 shows how you would join the *Prostate Problems* discussion list.

Once this initial mail has been sent the listserver will send you an e-mail, usually within a few minutes, asking you to confirm that you wish to join the list. This security feature ensures that other people cannot subscribe to lists on your behalf. Once you have replied to this mail you will be sent a further mail welcoming you to the group, explaining its purpose and providing administrative information, such as how to send messages to the list and how to unsubscribe (Fig. 6.2).

Though it may sound trivial, one of the most important things to understand about a discussion list is the difference between the address of the mailing list and the address of the listserver. Messages that relate to the administration of the list (joining, leaving etc) are sent to the listserver, whilst contributions to the discussion are sent to the list. Failing to comply with this basic rule results in 'unsubscribe' messages being sent to every list member. Box 6.2 shows how you would address a message to the *Prostate Problems* discussion list.

Box 6.2   Contributing to the *Prostate Problems* discussion list

Note that this message is sent directly to the list.

To:	prostate@listserv.acor.org
Subject:	Fish oil supplements
Text:	Does anyone know whether fish oil supplements …….

Once you have joined a list you need to ensure that you collect your e-mail on a regular basis if you wish to contribute to the debate. Posting a message that relates to a discussion that took place some weeks earlier will not endear you to other list members. You also need to be aware that some lists are very active and generate a significant number of messages. The *Prostate* list, for example, generates around 30 messages a week. If this becomes a problem, see if the list supports a digest option – here, you just get one message per day which contains all the messages – and/or a Web archive. If a list has such an archive you can just log on to this as and when time permits.

Newsgroups

Newsgroups are another way in which the Internet facilitates group-wide communication. Arranged on a subject-specific basis, newsgroups enable groups of like-minded people to come together to discuss matters of common interest. Whatever your interest – from learning about card tricks

<news://alt.magic.cardtricks>, to discussing the antics of the radio-folk *The Archers* <news://uk.media.radio.archers>, through to cooking for a diabetic patient <news://alt.food.diabetic> – you can be assured that a newsgroup exists to cater for your needs.

Newsgroups differ from discussion lists, however, in two important respects. Firstly, postings to a newsgroup are held on a news server; they are not copied to your personal electronic mailbox. Secondly, to read newsgroup messages you need an Internet Service Provider that offers a news-feed service. If your ISP does not offer this service, postings can be accessed via the Google service <http://groups.google.com/>. However, as a Web-based service this represents a far more time-consuming and cumbersome way of accessing newsgroup messages.

Internet newsgroups attract huge international audiences and as such are an excellent way to solicit opinions and seek advice. Many of them are also very active, generating a significant number of postings in a single day. For example, both the <news://alt.med.fibromyalgia> and the <news://alt.support.diabetes> newsgroups generate on average over 200 messages every day, from all parts of the connected world.

Arrangement of newsgroups

There are in excess of 35,000 newsgroups, organised into a hierarchical structure as shown in Table 6.1. For the health consumer, newsgroups in the <news://alt.support.> and the <news://sci.medicine.> hierarchies will be most

Table 6.1   Hierarchical arrangement of newsgroups

Category	Topic	Example
alt.	Alternative	alt.support.eating-disord
bionet.	Biology	bionet.genone.chromosomes
biz.	Business	biz.jobs.offered
comp.	Computers	comp.windows.news
humanities.	Humanities	humanities.classics
k12.	Education	k12.ed.science
misc.	Miscellaneous	misc.health.alternative
news.	News	news.admin.net-abuse.policy
rec.	Recreational	rec.gardens.roses
regional.	Regional	uk.people.support.epilepsy
sci.	Scientific	sci.med.diseases.osteoporosis
soc.	Society	soc.history.world.war.ii
talk.	Talk	talk.politics.mideast

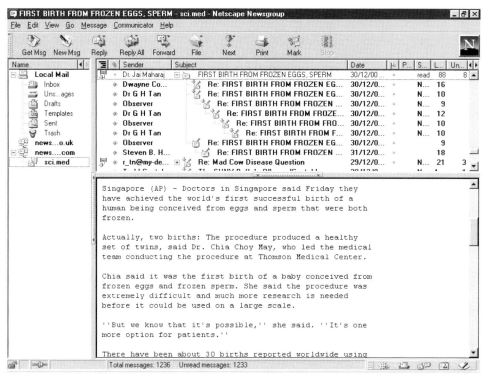

Fig. 6.3 Message threading

relevant, though newsgroups within the regional <news://uk.> and miscella-
neous <news://misc.> sections may also prove useful.

Messages sent to any newsgroup are arranged into threads, thus making it
easy to follow the original posting and the subsequent replies. Figure 6.3
shows a selection of message threads sent to the <news://sci.med> newsgroup.

Finding relevant newsgroups

The best way to identify a relevant newsgroup is to run a search against the
archive of newsgroup messages <http://groups.google.com> to see in which
forums previous discussions have taken place. For example, a search for 'lung
cancer' (Fig. 6.4) indicates that the newsgroups <news://alt.support.cancer>
and <news://sci.med.diseases.cancer> are the most appropriate groups to
carry postings on this topic.

Messages sent to these newsgroups can be accessed via the Google site.
However, a more efficient method is to log on to your local news server and
download all the messages posted to the groups you are interested in. Details
on how to do this using Netscape Navigator and Internet Explorer are provided
below (Box 6.3 and Box 6.4).

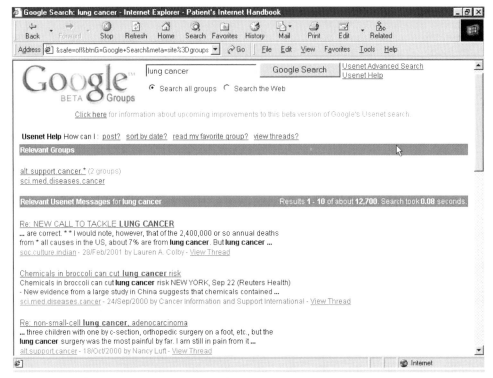

Fig. 6.4   Finding newsgroups via Google

Box 6.3   Accessing newsgroups via Netscape Navigator

Reading newsgroup messages via Netscape Navigator is a two-stage process. Firstly, you need to configure Netscape to access your Internet Service Provider's newsgroup server. Secondly, you need to specify which newsgroups you wish to subscribe to and then download the messages. Details on how to accomplish both tasks are provided below.

Step 1 – Configuring Netscape

- Open Navigator and select **Edit** ⟡ **Preferences** ⟡**Mail & Newsgroups** ⟡ **Newsgroup Servers** ⟡ **Add**

    In the Server dialogue box add the name of your newsgroup server, as supplied by your Internet Service Provider. This typically takes the form of news.name-of-service-provider. Thus NTLWorld customers use the address news.ntlworld.com, whilst Demon Internet customers log on to news.demon.co.uk.

Step 2 – Connecting and downloading newsgroup messages

- Open Netscape and select **Communicator** ⟡ **Newsgroups**
- Double-click on your news server address.

The first time you do this the server will download the names of the newsgroups to your browser. This may take some time (more than 5 minutes) – though you will only have to do this once.

- Click on **File** ◊ **Subscribe** and in the resulting dialogue box (Fig. 6.5) browse or search for the newsgroup(s) you wish to subscribe to.

- Once these have been identified, click on the **Subscribe** button.

  The hierarchical nature of newsgroups is shown by the ⌂ icon. Double-clicking on a folder will reveal the names. Figure 6.5 shows the newsgroups available in the alt.support.cancer hierarchy.

- To download the message headers – the one line piece of text that indicates what the posting is about – click on **File** ◊ **Get New Messages**. To view the contents of any message double-click on the header.

  If you have a dial-up connection and are being charged by the minute for the phone connection to your ISP, it makes sense to flag the records you wish to read and download these for reading offline.

  To flag a record click on the flag icon (Fig. 6.6) and select **File** ◊ **Get Flagged Messages**. Once the messages have been downloaded, you can cut your connection to your ISP. To read these messages, select **File** ◊ **Work Offline**. The flagged messages can now be read at your leisure.

- To send, or reply to any message, use the **New Message** and **Reply/ Reply to All** buttons on the Navigator toolbar.

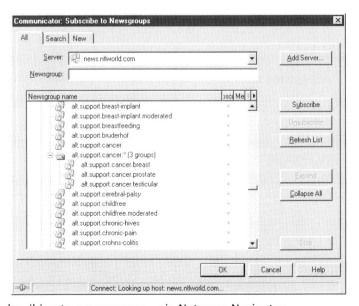

Fig. 6.5   Subscribing to a newsgroup – via Netscape Navigator

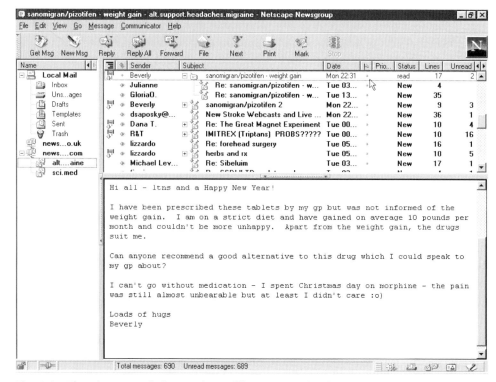

Fig. 6.6   Flagging records for reading offline – note the flag icon above the mouse pointer

Section 5 of this book also provides details of newsgroups for 100 common diseases and conditions.

Box 6.4   Accessing newsgroups via Internet Explorer/Outlook Express

Reading newsgroup messages via Internet Explorer is a three-stage process. Firstly, you need to define which newsreader you wish to use. Secondly you need to configure the newsreader to access your Internet Service Provider's newsgroup server. Thirdly, you need to specify which newsgroups you wish to subscribe to and download the messages. Details on how to accomplish these tasks are provided below.

Step 1 – Defining your newsreader

Internet Explorer can be configured to use any newsreader. In practice, however, it defaults to using Microsoft's Outlook Express.

- Open Explorer and select **Tools ◊ Internet Options ◊ Programs ◊ Newsgroups**. If you wish to use Outlook Express ensure that this is the selected programme.

Step 2 – Configuring Outlook Express

- Open Outlook Express and select **Tools ◊ Accounts ◊ News ◊ Add News**

  You are then prompted by the Internet Connection Wizard to supply various details, including the name of your newsgroup server, as supplied by your Internet Service Provider. This typically takes the form of news.name-of-service-provider. Thus NTLWorld customers use the address news.ntlworld.com, whilst Demon Internet customers log on to news.demon.co.uk.

Step 3 – Connecting and downloading newsgroup messages

- Open Outlook Express and double-click on the name of your news server.

  The first time you do this the server will download the names of the newsgroups to your browser. This may take some time (more than 5 minutes) – though you will only have to do this once.

- As you will not have yet subscribed to any newsgroups, Outlook Express gives you the option to view a list of the available newsgroups. Say **Yes** to this prompt and either browse, or search through, the list of available newsgroups. Figure 6.7 shows those newsgroups that have the string 'diabet' in the title. [The string 'diabet' was used as it would identify newsgroups that included either the term diabe**tes** or diabe**tic**.]

- To subscribe to any group, simply click on the **Subscribe** option.

- To download the messages in the newsgroup click on **Tools ◊ Download this newsgroup**. Outlook Express offers you the option to download just the message headers – the one line piece of text that indicates what the posting is about – or all the messages in their entirety. If you opt to view just the headers it is possible to mark the ones you want to read and collect these postings next time you log on.

- To send, or reply to any message, use the **Compose Message** and **Reply to Group/Reply to Authors** buttons on the Outlook Express toolbar.

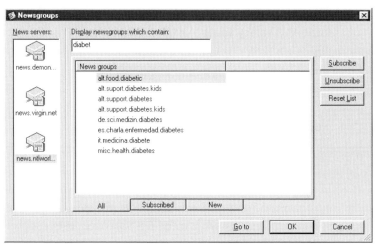

Fig. 6.7   Finding and subscribing to newsgroups via Outlook Express

Think before you speak

Before sending any message to a discussion list or Internet newsgroup consider carefully what you are going to say, and how much personal information (if any) you wish to disclose. Any message sent to a publicly accessible forum – such as a discussion list or newsgroup – may be seen and read by literally thousands of readers, from all over the globe.

Additionally, it is important to remember that most forums are archived and thus your message and any information you provide in it will be indexed and retrievable for many years. The Google server, for example, stores all newsgroup messages sent since 1995.

You also need to be conscious of how easy it is for your message to be forwarded to another list or newsgroup without your consent or knowledge. Thus even if you feel happy to share your concerns and emotions with a highly supportive newsgroup, would you necessarily feel the same way if that message found its way into other, less supportive forums?

When posting questions and replying to queries it is also important to remember the international nature of lists and newsgroups and to be aware that idioms and abbreviations may be meaningless or even offensive to readers in other parts of the world. The golden rule on all Internet communications is to write simply and clearly. If you think your message may be misunderstood, rephrase it.

Box 6.5 provides a summary of best-practice guidelines you should consider before contributing to a public discussion forum.

Box 6.5 Communicating via a public forum – good practice guidelines

- **Safeguard your identity**

  When posting a query about a specific medical condition to a discussion list or newsgroup be careful as to how much personal information you disclose. For example, ensure that your e-mail signature does **not** contain your full postal address.

  You may also wish to consider setting up a separate e-mail account, using a service such as Hotmail <http://www.hotmail.com> for contributing to these public forums. If you do this, you can use your default e-mail address for ordinary correspondence (writing to friends, family, colleagues etc.) and a more anonymous one for public forums. If anyone you normally write to stumbles across a message you sent to a newsgroup or discussion list they will be oblivious to the true identity of the sender.

- **Be polite**

  Many Internet users are put off from using newsgroups and discussion list through fear of receiving abusive mail in response to a question. In Internet parlance this is referred to as being 'flamed'.

  Although it is irritating to read postings that are either irrelevant to the discussion, or contain requests for information that has been provided countless times before, it is incumbent on all of us to remember that every Internet user is a 'newbie' at some point. A polite reply directing the user to a list of FAQs (Frequently Asked Questions) probably requires less effort than firing off an abusive e-mail and is more likely to result in the user remaining a member of that group.

- **Keep on-topic**

  A discussion forum focused on eating disorders <news://alt.support.eating-disord>, for example, is not the right place to post a question on, say, hip replacements. Use the information provided in this chapter to identify a more appropriate discussion list or newsgroup.

- **Check the FAQs and online archives**

  Most newsgroups and discussion lists keep a file of frequently asked questions (FAQs). Before posting a query to a public forum check the FAQ file to see if your question has already been answered. If the forum has a publicly searchable archive you should also consider searching this.

Conclusion

Discussion lists and newsgroups epitomise the best and worst aspects of the Internet. On the positive side such forums, particularly in the area of health, provide much-needed support and help. Though your doctor will be able to explain what your medical condition is and what can be done to treat it, it is unlikely that they will have had personal experience of the condition. As such, they will not be able to fully empathise with you or provide first-hand experience of how to cope with the illness. An online support group, however, will be populated almost entirely by people who have similar or identical conditions.

The value of discussion forums to health consumers has long been recognised by health professionals. Research that looked at ovarian cancer support groups concluded that such groups 'may become an important aspect of care to enhance quality of life' and that 'psychological interventions to support patients emotionally and to enhance their quality of life should therefore be considered an important complement to medical care'. For details see: <http://www.ncbi.nlm.nih.gov/entrez/query.fcgi?cmd=Retrieve&db=PubMed &list_uids=9250082&dopt=Abstract>.

On the other hand newsgroups (and to a lesser extent discussion lists) can also show the Internet in its very worst light. The tabloid-sponsored myth that the Internet only contains pornography is, to some extent, the consequence of a number of newsgroups, most notably in the <news://alt.sex.> hierarchy. Less sensationally, but of more relevance to health consumers, is the fact that much of what you read in a public discussion forum will be anecdotal and not based on hard, empirical evidence. One study that looked at the postings sent to the newsgroup <news://sci.med.pharmcy> concluded that around 20% of all the drug information provided here was deemed to be harmful. For details see: <http://www.ncbi.nlm.nih.gov/entrez/query.fcgi?cmd=Retrieve&db=PubMed &list_uids=9519647&dopt=Abstract>.

Consequently, as with all health information you find via the Internet, it is important that you discuss your findings with your doctor and other health professionals. As stressed throughout this book, the Internet should be used as a means of becoming better informed about your health so you can ask the 'right' questions when you visit your doctor. It should not lead you to become your own diagnostician, physician, or surgeon.

With these provisos in mind we would encourage all Internet users to make use of relevant discussion lists and newsgroups. They can be a useful source of information, be highly supportive, provide a sense of community and, perhaps best of all, be interesting and entertaining.

Your health and the Internet

Overview

Having provided an overview of how you can connect to the Internet and retrieve information appropriate to your needs, this next section adopts a more subject-oriented approach to health information on the Internet.

For many people the sole provider of health care is the NHS. In Chapter 7 we discuss how the NHS is using the Internet to disseminate information about the services it provides. Particular attention is paid to sources that allow consumers to compare one hospital with another. We also highlight a number of practical online services such as British Dental Association's 'Find-a-dentist' database and the NHS *Pharmacy Directory*.

Drug information is the focus of Chapter 8, where in addition to giving an overview of the key information sources, we discuss the role of online pharmacies and the potential dangers they pose.

Complementary and Alternative Medicine (CAM) is a topic of growing importance – some 5 million UK citizens used the services of a CAM practitioner in the past year – and in Chapter 9 we discuss some of the best Internet sources for this subject. Recognising that it would be virtually impossible to try to give an overview of information sources as they pertain to all types of CAM therapies, we have concentrated on the five principal disciplines – acupuncture chiropractic, herbal medicine, homeopathy and osteopathy. As with the chapter on the NHS, attention is paid to how the Internet can be used to find local, qualified practitioners.

The final chapter in this section looks at the information sources on the Internet pertaining to pregnancy, childbirth and infant care. Topics covered include tests and scans, giving birth, and immunisation. There is also information about a number of interactive tools, such as an ovulation calculator and an online birth plan.

CHAPTER 7

NHS services and the Internet

Introduction

The massive development of Internet-based services is leading to a society where many things are possible simply by 'pointing and clicking'. Services such as Internet shopping and banking – virtually unheard of two years ago – are now mainstream activities. Indeed, in the weeks leading up to Christmas 2000, the Internet book supply company Amazon <http://www.amazon.co.uk> dispatched more than 3.2 million items and had sales in excess of £640 million.

Just as businesses have moved to the Internet it is perhaps inevitable that health consumers should also look to this new medium to see what services are available. Certainly, there are services that offer online medical consultations. Cyberdocs <http://www.cyberdocs.com>, for example, enables anyone with an Internet connection (and a credit card) to obtain a private and confidential one-to-one consultation with a US-trained physician. In the UK e-med <http://www.e-med.co.uk> and Med4u <http://www.med4u.co.uk> offer similar services.

Anyone who wishes to use an online consultation needs to consider a number of issues. First, is a virtual consultation, where the doctor cannot actually see you, very useful? Secondly, what duty of care do these services provide? At the present time if you are treated in a way that is deemed to be negligent, formal action can be taken against the doctor or relevant health authority. These safeguards may not exist in an online environment.

In many ways, however, this type of service is still somewhat peripheral and outside the interest of most health consumers. In contrast, finding information about local NHS services, or trying to determine which hospital provides the best care, are more common concerns and ones we will focus on in this chapter.

NHS hospitals on the Web

The easiest way to determine what services your local hospital provides is to have a look at its Web site. In an attempt to provide easy access to this sort of information the NHS Executive have developed the NHS Web site

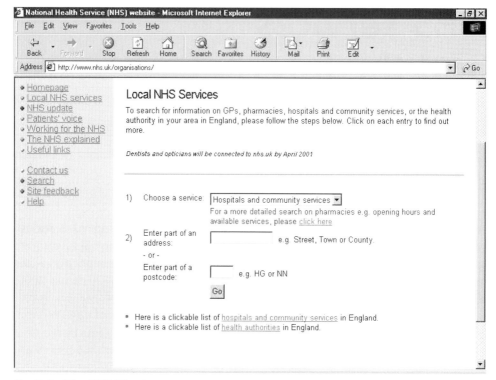

Fig. 7.1   The NHS Directory

<http://www.nhs.uk>. Central to this is a searchable directory of NHS services, which includes GPs and pharmacies as well as hospital and community trusts. Using the well-designed search screen (Fig. 7.1) you can readily identify services local to yourself.

Unfortunately, at the time of writing the only data you can access with regard to NHS hospitals is their postal address (along with an online map) and a telephone number. Even more frustrating, however, is the fact that though most hospitals have some sort of Web site, this information is not linked to the NHS site. Thus, though a search of the NHS Directory for hospitals in the Bath area will identify the Royal United Hospital and the Bath and West Community NHS Trust, you still need to use the search services discussed in Chapter 4 to find their respective Web sites.

Readers who make this extra step and find the Royal United Bath Web site <http://www.ruh-bath.swest.nhs.uk/> will be rewarded with a detailed profile of the hospital, annual reports, and up-to-date news. Similar information can be found on the Bath and West Community NHS Trust site <http://www.bwtrust.demon.co.uk/>.

Though there is a need for the NHS to make hospital Web sites more uniform – not least so that you can easily find information and compare it –

until this task is complete it seems absurd not to provide links to established sites via the NHS Directory.

Hospital statistics

Hospital statistics are another rich source of information. At one level they may simply serve to show how busy a particular hospital (or department) is, whilst figures that relate to performance, or the number of complaints it receives, give the consumer some idea as to how their local hospital compares with others.

For basic activity data the Hospital Activity pages, produced by the Department of Health, **<http://193.32.28.83/hospitalactivity/statistics/ 1999-00/hospital_activity_summary/y00.htm>** are a recommended starting point. Here, data on a range of services – number of critical care beds, Accident & Emergency attendances, supporting facilities etc – are available for every NHS Trust in the UK. Information relevant to your local Trust can be found by navigating a clickable map of the UK, or browsing through an alphabetical list of NHS Trusts. Figure 7.2 shows the summary activity data for the Royal Surrey County Hospital.

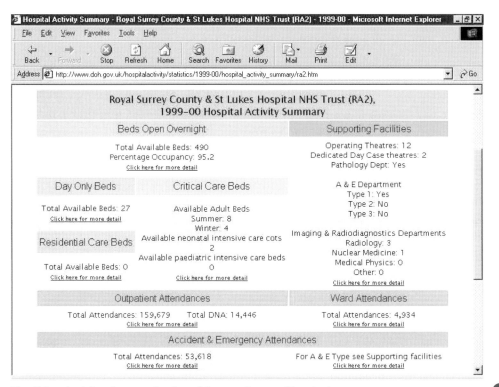

Fig. 7.2   Activity data at the Royal Surrey County Hospital

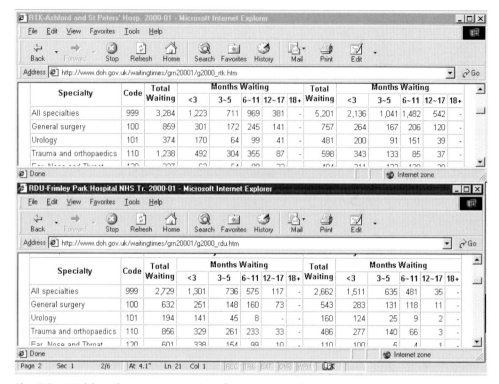

Fig. 7.3 Waiting times: a comparison between two hospitals

Waiting time data is another useful source of information – particularly if you are waiting for a hospital appointment and wish to see whether a referral to another hospital would expedite matters. Waiting time data is published by the Department of Health and is available at <http://www.doh.gov.uk/waitingtimes/>. At this site, data on both in-patient waiting times and waiting times for a first outpatient appointment are available for every English NHS Trust. Using the information presented here you can see, for example, that some 87 patients have been waiting for between 12 and 17 months at Ashford and St Peter's Hospital for a trauma/orthopaedic procedure, whereas at nearby Frimley Park Hospital only 33 patients have had to wait this long (Fig. 7.3).

Raw data on its own, however, does not tell the whole story. Crucially, it does not give you any indication as to the quality of the service you are likely to receive. For this information you need to consult the NHS Performance Indicators <http://www.doh.gov.uk/nhsperformanceindicators/>.

The Indicators set out NHS performance against 56 different measures, including cancer survival, patient complaints and deaths following surgery. For example, the figures show that 83% of patients diagnosed with breast cancer during the period 1991–93 in East Surrey survived for five years or more. In contrast, the survival rate was down to 64% for patients in the care of North Staffordshire Health Authority. Although it is true that crude comparisons can be misleading – specialist units, by virtue of the fact they undertake the more complex procedures, are always likely to have a higher death rate – these tables do enable patients to see how their local hospital is performing against a common benchmark. [Information from the sources described here was recently compiled into the *Sunday Times Good Hospital Guide*. This is available online at: <http://www.sunday-times.co.uk/news/pages/sti/2001/01/14/stipatcon01001.html>.]

Ready public access to this type of information is a most welcome development and one that certainly contributes to patient empowerment. However, in the wake of the scandal at the Bristol Royal Infirmary, where three doctors were found guilty of serious professional misconduct following the death of 29 babies and young children, and the news that surgeons at Alder Hey Hospital removed and retained children's organs without their parents' consent, the demand for even more information about a hospital's performance will grow.

In the United States a number of Health Boards already publish highly detailed hospital performance data on the Web. For example, at the New York

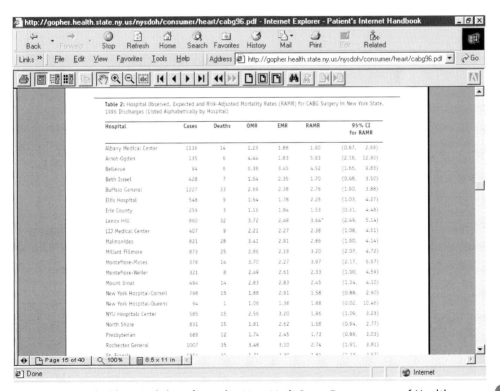

Fig. 7.4   Detailed hospital data from the New York State Department of Health

State Department of Health Web site <http://gopher.health.state.ny.us/nysdoh/consumer/heart/cabg96.pdf> anyone can access the risk-adjusted mortality rates – figures that take into account the complexity of cases – for each of the 32 hospitals that are licensed to undertake coronary artery bypass surgery. Using this data, patients can see that St Joseph's Hospital has the lowest risk-adjusted bypass surgery death rate (1.10 per 100 patients), while the Arnot Ogden Hospital has a less successful record of 5.93 deaths per 100 patients (Fig. 7.4). It can only be a matter of time before data of this kind is in the public domain in the UK.

GP surgeries on the Web

If you are trying to identify whether your local GP practice has a Web site, the UK GP Web site Database <http://www.internet-gp.com/gpsites/> is a useful starting point. Here, GP Web sites can be found by searching the database by location/or name of the practice. Alternatively, you can use a clickable map of the UK and browse the database by geographical area. Clicking on Surrey, for example, identifies (and links to) some twelve GP surgeries that have online Web sites. Information at the specific sites varies from practice to practice, though most provide details of the surgery hours, links to useful Web sites and a notice board where current information is posted.

Do not be surprised, however, if your local GP surgery is not identified through this database. It almost certainly means that your practice does not have a Web site. Indeed, out of an estimated 10,000 GP practices in the UK only about 450 have developed a Web site.

A more comprehensive directory of GP surgeries is available via the NHS Web site <http://www.nhs.uk>. As with the directory of hospitals, however, information provided here is limited to the name of the practice and its postal address.

Doctors on the Web

Having determined what local services are available, the next questions most health consumers want to ask are about the practising health professional. For example, you may wish to know whether your doctor has been the subject of any disciplinary action, or seek reassurance that s/he is receiving continuing medical education. Equally, if you are about to undergo some form of surgery for, say, breast cancer, it may be reassuring to determine whether or not the surgeon is a member of the British Association of Surgical Oncology <http://www.baso.org>. Beyond this it is fairly natural to try to find out how many times your surgeon has performed the operation and what the success rate was.

The obvious place to seek answers to questions of this nature is the Web site of the General Medical Council (GMC). The GMC are responsible for licensing all doctors who practise medicine in the UK.

Details on these individuals – some 190,000 of them – are contained in the *Medical Register*, which anyone can access on request. At the time of writing, however, this database was not accessible via the GMC Web site <http://www.gmc-uk.org/>. Anyone seeking this information is advised to telephone or write to the GMC. A note on the Web site advises visitors that an Internet version of the directory will be available 'early in 2001'.

A visit to the respective Web sites of the various Royal Colleges (independent, professional bodies that oversee the training and development needs of their members) proves equally disappointing. The Web sites of the Royal Colleges of Surgeons <http://www.rcseng.ac.uk/>, General Practitioners <http://www.rcgp.org.uk/>, Physicians <http://www.rcplondon.ac.uk/> and Anaesthetists <http://www.rcoa.ac.uk/> all provide useful information – but singularly fail to provide any information about their members.

Indeed, what these sources serve to show – more than anything else, in our opinion – is how little we can find out about the staff to whom we entrust our lives. Even when the GMC's *Medical Register* comes online, information will be limited to a basic biographical sketch – where and when the doctor qualified, and where they are currently working. As yet there seems little appetite for publishing information that will provide information about the *quality* of the work doctors perform.

In the United States, on the other hand, information of this kind is more readily available. The Annual Report of Cardiac Surgery in the state of New York, discussed above, not only shows how different hospitals compare, but also how individual surgeons compare. Using the Risk Adjusted Figures (which take into account the complexity of cases), patients can see which individual surgeons, identified by name, had the lowest death rate.

The State Medical Boards (the US equivalent to the GMC) also provide detailed information on the doctors that they have licensed. The Ohio Medical Board Licensee Profile Database <http://www.state.oh.us/med/> provides information on the length of time each physician has been licensed and how many Continuing Medical Education credits (ie how much training) they have acquired in the past 12 months. The Physicians Profile Database from the Massachusetts Board of Registration in Medicine <http://www.docboard.org/ma/df/masearch.htm> provides even more specific information, including malpractice data and details of any disciplinary actions ever taken against the physician (Fig. 7.5). Again, it can only be a matter of time before this type of information is available to anyone seeking information about doctors practising in the UK.

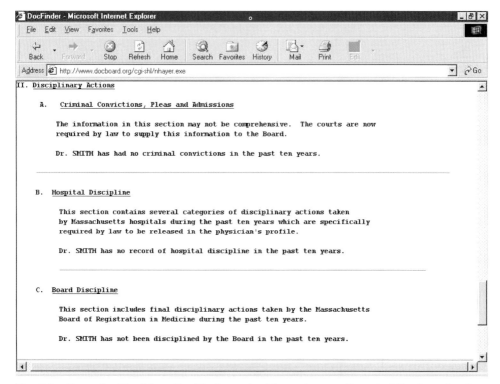

Fig. 7.5 Part of a Physicians Profile from the Massachusetts Board of Registration in Medicine

Dentists and opticians

The British Dental Association (BDA), the national body for UK dentists, has an impressive and highly useful Web site that includes a 'Find a dentist' database <http://www.bda-dentistry.org.uk/fad2/>. Each dentist who has agreed to be included in this resource has provided contact details, information about services provided (NHS, private etc) and details of facilities, such as wheelchair access and car parking.

Local dentists can be found by searching the database by postcode/address, as well by the specific features described here. Thus, it is possible to construct a search, for example, that identifies local dentists providing treatment on the NHS and weekend appointments. Figure 7.6 shows the full range of search options.

The BDA Web site also provides guidance on how to choose a dentist and gives useful tips on how to ensure the treatment you receive meets your needs. For example, if you have a fear of dentists the recommendation is to let the dentist know beforehand so that he or she can allow you extra time.

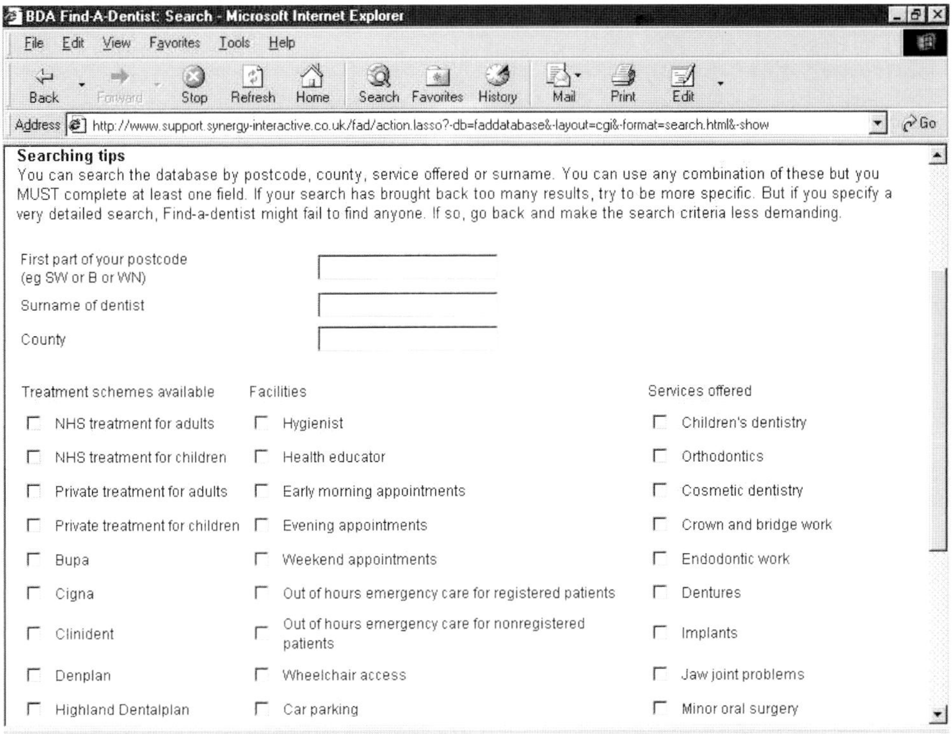

Fig. 7.6   Find-a-dentist at the BDA Web site

You can also use the Internet to identify local opticians. Unlike the dental profession, however, they have no central database you can access. In recognition of this a number of local authorities have pulled together this type of information – the Careline Centre in Wandsworth <http://www.careline.org.uk/> and the Lothian Opticians Database <http://www.edinburgh.gov.uk/Lothian_Health/Lothian_Opticians/opticians.html> are but two examples.

For a more national perspective you will need to use one of 'yellow pages' directory services such as Scoot <http://www.scoot.co.uk>, or Yell <http://www.yell.com>. Using the former site, a simple search for opticians in the Reading area identified 50 optical stores. As a minimum, each entry in the database contains basic contact details – telephone number, address and an online map to help you locate it. Companies who are prepared to pay for extra advertising space can also provide additional information, such as opening times and details of current special offers.

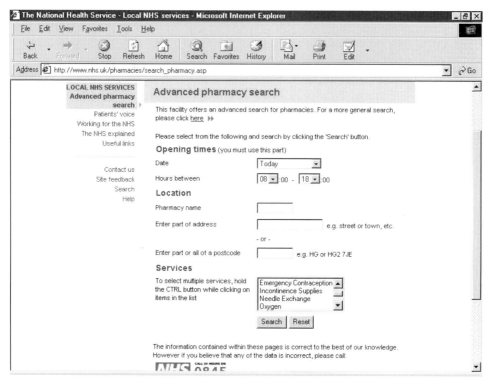

Fig. 7.7   Find a pharmacist – NHS gateway

Pharmacies

The NHS gateway site <http://www.nhs.uk> has a national directory of pharmacies. Unlike the hospital or GP surgery directories discussed above, the pharmacy directory contains a wealth of information, all of which has been indexed to facilitate easy retrieval. For example, in addition to being able to search the directory by postcode/address, you can add various other search criteria. These include the ability to search for pharmacies that offer specialist services – delivery service, emergency contraception etc – or those which open late. Figure 7.7 shows the full range of search options.

Information about the availability of drug information on the Internet and issues around buying drugs via this medium are discussed in Chapter 8.

Conclusion

From the comfort of your home it is already possible to find accurate and up-to-date information about many of the health services that are delivered through the NHS. Over the next few years even more information about these services – in particular, information that pertains to the quality of services – will be delivered through the Internet. In the wake of the tragedy at the Bristol Royal Hospital for Sick Children, it is perhaps fitting that this unit is one of the first in the UK to use the Internet to publish detailed reports on the work it performs <http://www.ubht.org.uk/bch/Reports/1998-9.htm>.

The recently published *NHS Plan – a plan for investment; a plan for reform* speaks of the importance of delivering patient-focused care and a commitment to ensuring that 'patients will have a real say in the NHS' and 'influence over the way it works' <http://www.nhs.uk/nationalplan/summary.htm>. If this objective is to be realised patients will need real data, presented in an accessible format, on how the NHS is performing. As this chapter has made clear, some of this information is already in the public domain, but some is not. Where there are omissions they need to be rectified. When public disclosure about health services and professionals becomes the norm the much-touted 'empowered patient' will become a reality.

CHAPTER 8

Drug information on the Internet

Introduction

Research shows that around 50% of patients fail to comply with the medication they are prescribed. The reasons for this are many, but a common recommendation for increasing compliance is to provide patients with more information about the drugs that are being prescribed. Obviously, the best forum for this is in the doctor–patient consultation, but if additional printed information is required, the Internet is the obvious place to look.

Through the Internet, health consumers (as well as health professionals) can find information on virtually all prescription drugs, including details of any reported adverse effects and usage instructions. This chapter will introduce you to best Web sources for this type of information. In addition to this we will look at the rise of online pharmacies and provide some practical guidelines about using them.

As with all the other subjects discussed in this book, it is important that you do not act upon any information you find on the Internet – particularly with regard to a drug you have been prescribed – without first discussing it with your doctor. Certainly, you should never unilaterally decide to stop taking a prescribed medicine. If, for example, you find information that concerns you about a drug you have been prescribed, make an appointment to see your doctor at the earliest opportunity to discuss this. Simply to stop taking the medication will almost certainly be more dangerous than any known side effect.

One should also be aware that drug data sheets (discussed below) are obliged to report all known adverse effects and contraindications, no matter how rarely or infrequently they occur. As a result, you can sometimes get a misleading impression as to how safe (or dangerous) a particular drug may be. Again, the best advice is to discuss these concerns with your doctor and ask what the level of risk is.

The Internet helps all of us to become more informed about our health – it does not, however, make us a doctor or a pharmacist.

With these provisos firmly in mind, it is time to open up our browsers and see what drug information we can find on the Internet.

Drug information – the key sources

In this section we describe four key resources for identifying accurate and up-to-date drug information. In many ways the sites described here can be seen hierarchically. Starting with the more general source, the Electronic Medicine's Compendium will provide you with the core information about any UK licensed drug. For more detailed information – though with a US bias – you should progress to the US Pharmacopoeia.

If you wish to take your investigations further, search the drug database at PharmInfo. Here you will be able to find original peer-reviewed articles about specific drugs. Finally, we come to the British National Formulary. Aimed at health professionals this source contains similar information to that found in the data sheet compendiums, but from a more critical viewpoint. It also offers a sophisticated search interface that allows you to identify how one drug interacts with another.

Each source has its own strengths and which you use will, to a large extent, depend upon your information requirements.

Electronic Medicine's Compendium

<http://emc.vhn.net/public>

The Electronic Medicine's Compendium (eMC) provides electronic versions of the official Patient Information Leaflet (PIL) and the Summary of Product Characteristics (SPC) for each of the 2500 medicines licensed for use in the UK. PILs, produced by the pharmaceutical companies, are the leaflets that accompany every prescription medicine. SPCs contain similar information, though the intended audience is the health professional. Via the eMC site health consumers can get access to both these information sources.

To find information about a specific drug you simply enter its name (or part of it) into the search box and hit the 'Return' key (Fig. 8.1). Usefully, this index of drugs includes both the product name (the commercial name assigned by the manufacturers) and the generic name. For example, information about the drug Adizem (typically prescribed for someone with angina) can be found by this name, or by its generic name, diltiazem.

Once the drug has been identified in the database you are presented with the opportunity to view either the SPC or the PIL. If you opt to view the former you can read about known contraindications (ie when the drug should not be taken), possible side effects and details of how the drug should be taken and stored. The PIL provides much the same data, but in a more accessible question and answer format. Typical questions posed (and answered) include 'What should I do if I forget to take my medicine?', and 'How should I take the

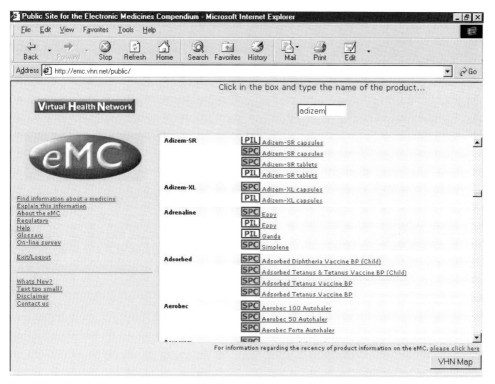

Fig. 8.1 Searching the Electronic Medicine's Compendium

medicine?'. Every SPC and PIL indicates when it was written and last updated.

To use the eMC site you need to complete an online registration form. Though this is compulsory, no charges are levied to use the service.

US Pharmacopoeia – advice for the patient

<http://www.intelihealth.com/IH>

The US Pharmacopoeia (USP) is another useful source of drug information. Compiled by the US Pharmacopeial Convention, data in the USP is derived from a peer-review consensus process that involves 800 volunteers serving on expert advisory panels.

Information in the USP as it pertains to a specific drug can be found by searching the database by generic or trade name. As this is a US source, however, be aware that a drug licensed for use in the UK may have a different name in the US. In the light of this fact it is advisable to search the USP using the drug's generic name. [Note, each PIL and SPC from the eMC site discloses the drug's generic name.]

Though in many ways this source provides similar information to that available via the eMC site, the overall impression we gained was that information in the USP is more detailed. For example, the UK data sheet for the anti-depression drug Seroxat (generic name paroxetine) advises the patient to discuss with their doctor the suitability of taking this drug if they are pregnant or might become pregnant soon. Though this is good advice – and one that is repeated in the USP – the American data sheets provide additional, supporting, information:

> One study looked at the babies of 97 women who took paroxetine either at the beginning of pregnancy or through the entire pregnancy. This study found no harmful effects of paroxetine on the babies. However, more study is needed to be sure that paroxetine is safe to use during pregnancy.

Similarly, UK consumers are warned 'not to take Seroxat if you are taking monomine oxidase inhibitors (MAOIs)'. Again, the same recommendation is provided in the USP, though on this occasion we are told what will happen if these drugs are taken in combination:

> You may develop confusion, agitation, restlessness, stomach or intestinal symptoms, sudden high body temperature, extremely high blood pressure, severe convulsions, or the serotonin syndrome.

The USP also includes images of the various pills in the database – thus providing visual reassurance that the information you have found relates to the drug you have been prescribed. This is particularly useful as so many drugs have very similar sounding names.

Pharminfo

<http://www.pharminfo.com>

If you wish to identify even more information about a specific drug, the database compiled by the team at Pharminfo is highly recommended. The drug database – which like all the other sources discussed here can be browsed or searched by either trade or generic name – provides links to original journal articles that discuss the effects and adverse effects of specific medications.

Continuing with the example of the anti-depressant drug paroxetine, a search of the Pharminfo database identifies seven articles. One of these focuses specifically on the safety of this drug for breastfeeding mothers <http://www.pharminfo.com/pubs/druginfoline/druginfo2_318c.html>, whilst a more general article considers the effectiveness of this drug. Interestingly, though this latter article discusses the clinical trials that demonstrated the efficacy of this drug in managing depression, it also reveals that 'in world-wide clinical trials, 21% of patients withdrew from paroxetine treatment because of adverse effects' <http://www.pharminfo.com/pubs/msb/paxil.html>.

British National Formulary

<http://www.bnf.org>

The British National Formulary (BNF) provides UK health professionals with 'authoritative and practical information on the selection and clinical use of medicines'. Published by the British Medical Association and the Royal Pharmaceutical Society of Great Britain, the BNF is the drug source most doctors and pharmacists refer to.

In recent months the information contained in the BNF has migrated to the Web. And, though in practice most health professionals still use the printed source (conveniently designed to fit into the doctor's pocket), the Web version

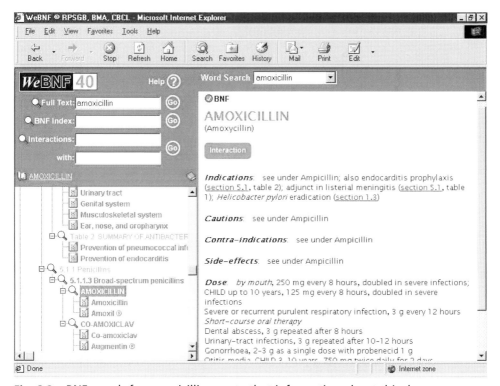

Fig. 8.2   BNF search for amoxicillin – note that information about this drug appears in various sections of the BNF

contains all the information that is available in the printed version, with the added functionality of full-text searching and retrieval.

Various options are available for finding information on a specific drug within the BNF. You can, for example, browse through the contents list and select any chapter you are interested in. Though in most cases this approach is of little use if you are looking for a specific drug, it may be valuable if you are looking for an overview of the drug options available for a particular body system – such as the cardiovascular or respiratory system.

The second and more practical option is to search the BNF. When doing this you can elect to search the entire text, or if this yields too many hits, you can search the book index. Figure 8.2 shows the results of a full-text search for the drug amoxicillin. Because this antibiotic can be used to treat a range of bacterial infections – from ulcers through to bronchitis and gonorrhoea – the information in the BNF is arranged to facilitate easy access to the most relevant section.

Finally, there is the option to perform an 'interactions search'. Here, you can enter the name of a drug and identify which other drugs it interacts with. Using this feature to look for information about sildenafil (the generic name for Viagra) you can quickly see that there are a significant number of other

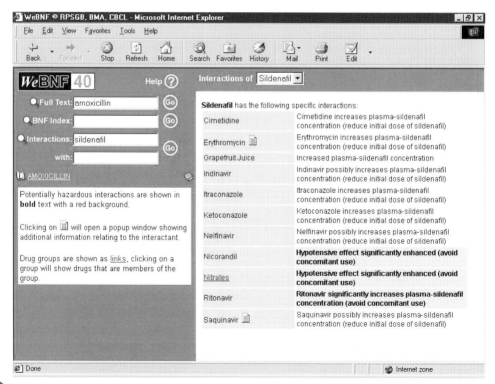

Fig. 8.3   An interactions search of the BNF

drugs that it interacts with (Figure 8.3). Potentially hazardous interactions are shown in bold text with a red background.

Information in the BNF is presented in a clear and consistent way, enabling the doctor to quickly find (and absorb) the key messages in terms of dosage requirements, known contraindications, side effects, etc. The BNF also adopts a more critical view than that presented in the official PILs. For example, information in the BNF about the drug paroxetine makes it clear that during initial treatment of panic disorder, 'there is potential for worsening of panic symptoms'. The relevant PIL makes no reference to this possibility.

The BNF also provides very practical guidance. Thus before prescribing nystatin (used to treat fungal infections) doctors are alerted to the fact this treatment will stain clothes yellow. Though this is hardly life threatening, this sort of information may be useful to know.

It should be stressed, however, that the BNF site is aimed at health professionals. Though the information is presented clearly, no attempt is made to 'translate' any of the material into a more patient-friendly language. Similarly, it does not spell out things that are obvious to the health professional. Thus, whereas the BNF might cite hyperkalaemia as a possible side effect of triamterne, it would not go on to include arrhythmias, since the professional will know that the latter is a consequence of the former.

If, however, you are prepared to accept these limitations you will discover that the BNF is a rich and authoritative source of drug information.

[Note: The BNF site makes extensive use of Java. Consequently, to use this site you must be using a Java-enabled Web browser, such as Netscape 3.0 or above or Internet Explorer 3.0 or above.]

Online pharmacies

Having determined what drug information is available online the next logical question is to determine to what extent drugs can be ordered (and dispensed) online.

The first thing to say is that obtaining prescription medicines via the Internet is possible, legal and safe – providing your prescription has been properly authorised by a registered doctor and the virtual pharmacy has been licensed. In the UK the Royal Pharmaceutical Society has approved two such pharmacies – Pharmacy2u and Allcures – discussed below.

If, however, you purchase drugs without a proper prescription, or from an unlicensed outlet, you are exposing yourself to unnecessary dangers. Selling prescription drugs is big business and, not surprisingly, there are rogue sites on the Internet that will sell drugs to consumers even when the need is dubious and the danger of an adverse reaction relatively high. Many of these Web sites prescribe once the consumer has completed an online questionnaire, thus bypassing the traditional safeguard of a face-to-face consultation with the health professional.

Only last year (2000) the US Food and Drug Administration (FDA) reported the case of a 52-year-old male who died after taking Viagra. In this instance the drug had been purchased over the Internet after the consumer had completed an online questionnaire. The drug had been prescribed even though the consumer had had episodes of chest pain and a family history of heart disease <http://www.fda.gov/fdac/features/2000/100_online.html>.

In addition to the dangers of obtaining drugs that may be unsuitable, there are other risks such as the drug being out of date (all drugs have a best-use-by date), or the supplier either failing to deliver or delivering the wrong product. This latter problem is particularly pertinent if ordering from an overseas site where different brand names may exist.

Box 8.1 provides a quick reference guide to buying prescription medicines online.

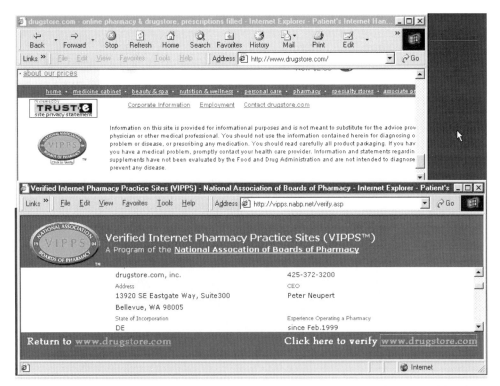

Fig. 8.4   The VIPPS seal of approval at the drugstore.com site – authenticated by the VIPPS authentication system

Box 8.1 **Buying prescription medicines online – a consumer safety guide**

- Obtain a prescription from your doctor. Do not buy online from sites that offer to prescribe a medicine without first undertaking an examination by a qualified doctor.

- Place your prescription with a UK-based service. In the event of any problem (medication not turning up etc) you will have the full consumer rights legislation to draw upon.

- Check that the site has been approved by the Royal Pharmaceutical Society (RPS). At the moment the only way to do this is to contact the RPS and ask them. In the US the National Association of Boards of Pharmacy have created a VIPPS (Verified Internet Pharmacy Practice Sites) seal of approval <http://www.nabp.net>. If a US online pharmacy displays this seal the user can click on it and independently verify that the service has been approved (Fig. 8.4). Hopefully, a similar system will be developed in the UK.

- Ensure that the site has a contact telephone number (test it to check that they answer) and a postal address.

- Ensure that the site has a clear privacy policy.

- Ensure that the site uses secure encryption technologies (see Chapter 3) before you pass on details of your medical history and credit card.

- If you are concerned about any issue regarding prescription drugs, consult your GP.

Online dispensing

As mentioned above, however, there are several genuine online pharmacies that offer the same high-quality service you would get from your local pharmacist, along with the added benefits of online ordering and potentially lower costs.

Allcures

<http://www.allcures.com>

Allcures.com are the UK's first full-service online pharmacy, offering both NHS and private prescriptions and a full range of over-the-counter medicines. As

---

Box 8.2   Ordering prescriptions from Allcures.com

1. Register on the Allcure site <http://www.allcures.com>.

2. Complete a simple online form, disclosing the prescription number and confirming the address to which the prescription should be sent. If you are not exempt from prescription charges it is at this point that you pay for your prescription, via a secure online credit card transaction.

3. Post your prescription to Freepost, Allcures.com – at the present time this cannot be sent electronically. If you are exempt from prescription charges a photocopy of your exemption certificate should be enclosed with your order.

4. Await delivery. Allcures undertake to deliver your prescription – completely free of charge – to any UK address, within three days of receiving the prescription.

---

with any high street pharmacy, the Allcures outlet does not write out prescriptions – you still need to get the prescription from your doctor. Box 8.2 describes the steps you need to take to get a prescription fulfilled via the Allcures Web site.

Pharmacy2U

<http://www.pharmacy2u.co.uk>

Pharmacy2U provides a similar service to Allcures, though at the time of writing they were unable to fulfil NHS prescriptions. Private prescriptions are placed through a Freepost service, and again no charge is made for prescription delivery.

Online dispensing – analysis

Unless you happen to live a long way away from a pharmacy, or never have the time to visit one when they are open, it is difficult to see what real benefits online pharmacies deliver. As you still have to get your prescription from your doctor, it will almost certainly be more convenient to pop into your local pharmacy and get them to fulfil the prescription. Moreover, if you need the medication now, then a three-day wait for the medication to arrive is hardly acceptable.

In the not-too-distant future, however, it is likely that doctors and nurse prescribers will be able to write out a prescription electronically (an e-prescription). When this happens you will simply designate which pharmacy you wish to use – a local, or a virtual one – and the prescription request will be sent electronically. Though you will still have to wait for the order to be fulfilled, in the case of repeat prescriptions etc the online pharmacy may be the more convenient option.

How quickly this scenario will come to pass is difficult to say. In the US e-prescriptions are already written and accepted. Companies such as e-Physician <http://ephysician.com> and I-Scribe <http://www.iscibe.com> have developed handheld prescribing devices that allow the doctor to write a prescription, view the patient's prescribing history and send signed prescriptions wirelessly to any registered pharmacy in the US. How quickly the UK will follow this lead remains to be seen. However, the passing of the Electronic Communications Act 2000, which makes digital signatures legally admissible, is an important first step.

Conclusion

Drug information on the Internet is arguably the most contentious and difficult issue health professionals and regulatory bodies have to cope with. Indeed, the legislation that prohibits pharmaceutical companies from advertising directly to UK consumers seems increasingly meaningless at a time when Internet drug advertising is so prevalent and online drug purchasing a reality.

The Internet, as this chapter has demonstrated, is a rich source of information about prescription medicines. Using the sources discussed here we can all find out more about the various pills, creams and lotions that we have been prescribed. This information, however, does not make us qualified doctors or pharmacists. Instead, we should be using this material to help us to formulate meaningful questions to take to our GP. When we can do this effectively and participate actively in the doctor/patient consultation, then patient empowerment will be more than just a slogan.

CHAPTER 9

Complementary and alternative medicine on the Internet

Introduction

A recent House of Lords Select Committee report into complementary and alternative medicine (CAM) opened with the statement that 'the use of CAM is widespread and increasing across the developed world' <http://www.parliament.the-stationery-office.co.uk/pa/ld199900/ldselect/ldsctech/123/12301.htm>.

Figures for the UK certainly support this view. It has been estimated that up to 5 million UK citizens consulted a CAM practitioner in the past year and that, overall, 1 in 5 people have at some point used CAM. Furthermore, it has been reported that some 40% of GPs have referred their patients to CAM practitioners.

The reasons for the rise in popularity of CAM are numerous. Dissatisfaction with conventional medicine, coupled with a desire to seek alternative therapies, is the most obvious explanation for this phenomenon. Other factors, however, are also playing a part. These include a growing scepticism towards science and medicine (fuelled by the BSE/CJD, and the GM food debate) and a cultural one, where people increasingly want to feel that they are in control of all aspects of their lives, including health.

Given the interest in CAM it is hardly surprising that the Internet is awash with information on these topics. A simple AltaVista search for 'alternative medicine' identifies some 237,000 Web pages. Unfortunately for the information-seeker the quality of information on this subject is extremely variable. At one end of the spectrum you will find high-quality studies, such as the Consensus Reports on acupuncture published by the US National Institutes of Health (NIH) <http://odp.od.nih.gov/consensus/cons/107/107_intro.htm> and the Alternative Medicine Fact Sheets, published by the National Center for Complementary and Alternative Medicine (NCCAM) <http://nccam.nih.gov/nccam/fcp/factsheets/>. At the other end, a whole gambit of miracle cures and unproven techniques are waiting to ensnare the unwary surfer. These include claims that cancer (all forms) can be cured by use of an electrical 'zapper' <http://www.drclark.ch/cancer/canc_frame.htm> and that crystal therapy can be used to treat a variety of mental, emotional and physical problems <http://www.spacemagic.com/crystals.html>. The need to appraise judiciously all the information you find is essential, and will be discussed further in Chapter 11.

Recognising that it would be virtually impossible to try to give an overview of the information sources as they pertain to all types of CAM therapies, we have concentrated instead on the principal five disciplines – acupuncture, chiropractic, herbal medicine, homeopathy and osteopathy. For each of these we will highlight key sources, focusing on those Web sites that provide details of current research and give practical information, such as how to find a qualified practitioner. To start, however, we will provide a quick guide to some of the best umbrella-type CAM resources.

CAM on the Web

Gateway sites

All of the evaluated gateway services, discussed in Chapter 4, provide links to a range of high-quality sites that focus on CAM. Of particular note is the alternative medicine section within MEDLINE*plus* <http://www.nlm.nih.gov/medlineplus/alternativemedicine.html>. Here, information pertaining to ongoing clinical trials, current research and the latest news about CAM is all conveniently accessible from one page. Most importantly, information at this site is very up-to-date. Looking at this site in late January 2001 there was a link to an Associated Press story that discussed recently published research (*Lancet* 2001; **357**: 251–56) which showed that the nutritional supplement glucosamine sulfate could be the first treatment to slow the progression of osteoarthritis.

MEDLINE*plus*, however, only indexes around fifteen or so CAM Internet resources. For a more comprehensive gateway site the New York Online Access to Health (NOAH) service is highly recommended <http://www.noah-health.org/english/alternative/alternative.html>. Here, Internet resources are categorised both by the specific form of CAM – acupuncture, aromatherapy, reflexology etc – and by disease. Using this latter approach, you can readily find information about the use of CAM in managing conditions such as AIDS, asthma and multiple sclerosis (Fig. 9.1).

NOAH is a joint project between the City University of New York, the Metropolitan New York Library Council, the New York Academy of Medicine and the New York Public Library. As with all gateway sites no guarantees are given as to the quality of the information on the sites this service links to. That said, however, the NOAH service aims to provide 'high quality full-text health

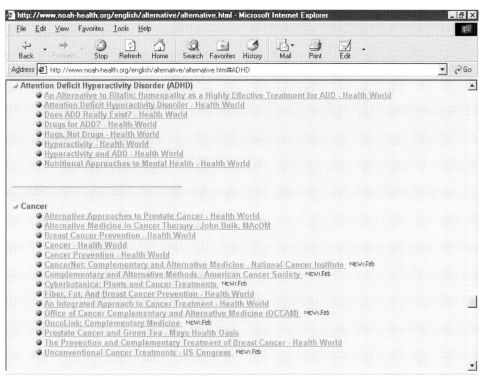

Fig. 9.1   New York Online Access to Health (NOAH)

information for consumers that is accurate, timely, relevant and unbiased' – and to help realise this it has adopted a clear (and publicly accessible) Web site selection policy <http://www.noah-health.org/english/collection.html>.

Current research

The CAM Citation Index, discussed in Chapter 5, is the best source for identifying ongoing research into the effectiveness of complementary and alternative therapies <http://nccam.nih.gov/nccam/resources/cam-ci/>. Journals indexed by this database include the *British Medical Journal* (*BMJ*) <http://www.bmj.com> and the *Alternative Medicine Review* <http://www.thorne.com/altmedrev/>. Both these titles have a Web presence, and in the case of the *BMJ* all articles are available free of charge in full text. The Web developers at the *BMJ* have also introduced a 'Collected Resources' section. From the Complementary Medicine page <http://www.bmj.com/cgi/collection/complementary_medicine> you can access every article the *BMJ* has published on this topic in the past three years.

Reports

An excellent overview of CAM has been produced by the Department of Health, in association with the Foundation for Integrated Medicine, the NHS Alliance and the National Association of Primary Care <http://www.doh.gov.uk/cam/index.htm>. This document – *Complementary Medicine: information for primary care clinicians* – provides a brief synopsis of individual therapies, describes what qualifications CAM practitioners should possess, and considers which patients or conditions would benefit most from the CAM therapies. Based on the published evidence, acupuncture, for example, is considered suitable for patients with chronic low back pain or those who suffer from migraines or dysmenorrhoea.

The report also includes the names and addresses of the various official bodies that regulate (or at least oversee) the use of CAM in the UK. Thus, though the practice of aromatherapy is not regulated in the UK – anyone can set up in business and claim to be a practitioner – this document advises that any NHS professional who wishes to offer this form of therapy should have trained to AOC standard (Aromatherapy Organisations Council). It makes sense therefore, if you are thinking of using an aromatherapist, to check that your practitioner has AOC approval. [*Note: This report has been published in PDF format. See Chapter 3 for details on how to download a PDF viewer, such as Adobe Acrobat.*]

Another interesting report into CAM has been published by the House of Lords Select Committee <http://www.parliament.the-stationery-office.co.uk/pa/ld199900/ldselect/ldsctech/123/12301.htm>. This comprehensive report provides information on the growth in the use of CAM in the UK, considers to what extent patients are satisfied by the treatment they receive and examines the general state of the CAM evidence base.

Having considered the more general Web sites we will now turn our attention to Internet resources that focus on the five key CAM disciplines.

Acupuncture

As highlighted in the Department of Health report (discussed above) there is a growing body of evidence that for certain conditions acupuncture can be an effective form of treatment. This evidence-based research can be accessed through the Cochrane Database of Systematic Reviews <http://www.update-software.com/cochrane/cochrane-frame.html>. A simple search for 'acupuncture' (conducted early in 2001) identified a number of reviews, including one that considered the role acupuncture can play in inducing labour and another that looked at the efficacy of this therapy for asthma sufferers.

Though in the UK acupuncture is not yet licensed, two bodies – the British

Medical Acupuncture Society (BMAS) and the British Acupuncture Council (BAcC) – are working hard to introduce professional standards.

BMAS is an association of medical practitioners (mainly doctors) interested in acupuncture. Via the BMAS Web site <http://www.medical-acupuncture.co.uk/index.shtml> you can learn about 'hot topics', get access to selected articles from the *Acupuncture in Medicine* journal, and identify a registered practitioner in your locality (Fig. 9.2). As this directory only lists fully accredited members of the British Medical Acupuncture Society, holding the Diploma of Medical Acupuncture, it represents an excellent source for finding a qualified practitioner.

The BAcC is a similar organisation, though one whose membership tends to be drawn from the ranks of physiotherapists and nurses rather than doctors. The BAcC strongly believes that anyone who wishes to provide acupuncture treatment 'should undertake an extensive training of at least two years full-time (or the part-time equivalent) *irrespective* of their prior western medical training'.

At the BAcC Web site <http://www.acupuncture.org.uk/> you will find similar types of information to that published on the BMAS site, including a

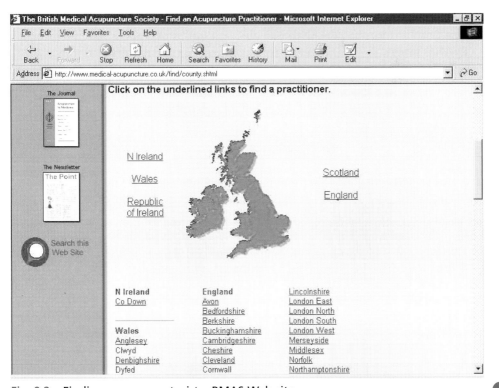

Fig. 9.2   Finding an acupuncturist – BMAS Web site

link to their journal, the *European Journal of Oriental Medicine* <http://www.ejom.co.uk/frame.html>. Though this site is painfully slow to access, if you persevere you will be rewarded with a significant online archive of articles, many of which are available in full-text free of charge.

Less impressive (and less convenient) is the section on finding a local BAcC practitioner. Unlike the BMAS site, visitors here are advised to phone or email the Council for a list of local, qualified practitioners.

Chiropractic

In contrast to acupuncturists, chiropractors are regulated by statute in the UK. Anyone who describes himself/herself as a chiropractor must register with the General Chiropractic Council (GCC) and abide by its regulations. As with any regulatory body, individuals can be struck off for malpractice.

The GCC Web site <http://www.gcc-uk.org/> includes background information about chiropractic as well as providing an online directory of all UK-registered chiropractors. This directory can be browsed alphabetically (by surname) or by county. Each entry in the register includes the name and contact details of the practitioner and information about when they regis-tered. As a list of practitioners by county can generate a significant number of entries, the 'Find on Web page' feature within the Web browser [Edit ◊ Find] can be used to identify quickly those who are based in a more specific location.

Further information about this form of treatment can be found in the *BMJ*'s 'ABC of Complementary Medicine' series <http://bmj.com/cgi/content/full/ 319/7218/1176> and at the Web site of the World Federation of Chiropractic <http://www.wfc.org/english/facts.html>.

Herbal medicine

The House of Lords Report into CAM defined herbal medicine as 'a system of medicine that uses various remedies derived from plant and plant extracts to treat disorders and maintain good health'.

In the UK, the British Herbal Medicine Association (BHMA) <http://www.ex.ac.uk/phytonet/bhma.html> exists to 'advance the science and practice of herbal medicine'. In support of this objective the BHMA pub-lishes the British Herbal Pharmacopoeia which details quality standards for 169 herbs commonly used in the UK for the preparation of botanical drugs. Though information about this publication is available on the Web <http://info.ex.ac.uk/phytonet/pubs.html> the full-text of this compendium is not.

Concern about the safety of herbals is an important issue and one that the European Scientific Co-operative on Phytotherapy has focused on. Information

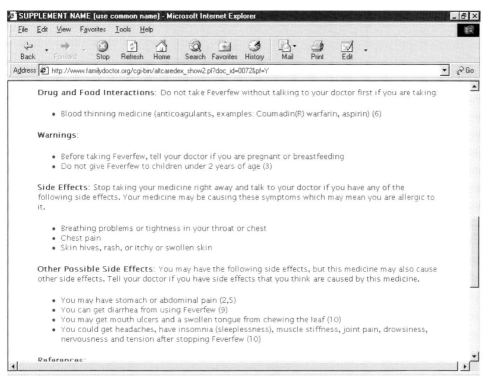

Fig. 9.3   Herbal and Alternative Remedies Database

about their work is available on the Web <http://info.ex.ac.uk/phytonet/welcome.html> – though the reporting of adverse reactions, and access to this data, is restricted to health professionals.

For information on a specific herbal one of the best sources is the Herbal and Alternative Remedies Database, hosted by the American Academy of Family Physicians <http://www.familydoctor.org/cgi-bin/altcaredex_search2.pl>. Each entry in the database provides details of the herbal, gives advice you should heed before using, and highlights known and possible side effects. Figure 9.3 shows part of the entry for the herbal feverfew.

Homeopathy

The Web site of the British Homeopathic Association <http://www.trusthomeopathy.org/> contains the usual mix of information about the association and background information on the practice of homeopathy. It also provides a searchable database of homeopathic doctors. Everyone included in this database is a member of the Faculty of Homeopathy, has a recognised medical qualification and has undertaken subsequent training in homeopathy at one of the five postgraduate homeopathic teaching centres approved by the Faculty. This database can be searched by postcode, city or county.

Another useful information source is the British Homeopathic Library (BHL) <http://dspace.dial.pipex.com/hom-inform/> and more specifically their Hom-Inform Database <http://hominform.soutron.com/> which provides an index to the published literature (books and journal articles) on homeopathy. Though the references are not available in full-text online, almost all of them are held by the BHL at their headquarters in Glasgow. Physical access to the library is open to anyone – daily fee £5.00, annual membership £25.00 per year – and a document supply service is also available. For details of current prices for this service see: <http://dspace.dial.pipex.com/hom-inform/bhl_sales.html>.

Finally, the *British Homeopathic Journal*, the leading UK publication in this field, is also available online. Though access to the full-text articles is restricted to those who subscribe to the printed copy, anyone can access the tables of contents for all issues published since April 1998, and set up an alerting service to receive by e-mail all subsequent tables of contents. For details see: <http://www.stockton-press.co.uk/bhj/>.

Osteopathy

Like chiropractors, osteopaths are statutorily regulated in the UK. The body responsible for regulating this profession is the General Osteopathic Council (GOC), whose Web site <http://www.osteopathy.org.uk/> provides a wealth of information about osteopathy, including fact-sheets, details of recent published research and a database of registered practitioners. Searchable by name, town, county and postcode this database provides contact details of registered osteopaths, including e-mail addresses where available. Figure 9.4 shows a selection of osteopaths who are based in Guildford.

The GOC site also provides a link to their official publication, *The Osteopath*. This, however, is not available online, unlike the *Journal of the American Osteopathic Association*, published by the American Osteopathic Association <http://www.am-osteo-assn.org/Publications/JAOA/jaoa.htm>. Though this title is aimed at practising osteopaths, anyone interested in this topic will find something that appeals amongst the selection of articles that this site makes freely available.

One other interesting Web resource on this topic is the Michigan State University College of Osteopathic Medicine's *Visualisation of Osteopathic Principles and Practice* <http://hal.bim.msu.edu/>. Again, aimed at health professionals, this site provides an interactive guide (complete with video clips) to help professionals 'learn and review concepts and skills necessary to successfully diagnose and treat dysfunction of the musculoskeletal system'.

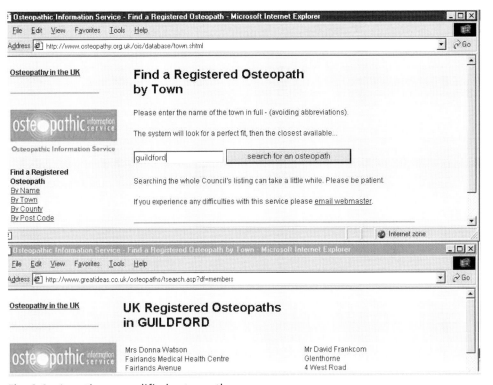

Fig. 9.4   Locating a qualified osteopath

Though the full product is only available on CD-ROM, the sample pages on the Web provide a useful insight into osteopathy.

Quackery and frauds

As alluded to in the introduction, some of the information on the Internet about complementary and alternative medicine is highly dubious and unproven. Two sites that try to draw consumers' attention to this fact (and highlight examples of this type of mis-information) are Quackwatch and the National Council Against Health Fraud (NCAHF).

Quackwatch <http://www.quackwatch.com>, set up by retired psychiatrist Dr Stephen Barrett, provides practical advice on how to identify rogue sites – for example, those that promote a single therapy that can cure all diseases – and, more generally, advocates the need to be wary of some alternative treatments <http://www.quackwatch.com/01QuackeryRelatedTopics/altway. html>.

The NCAHF <http://www.ncahf.org/> is a private voluntary health agency that also focuses upon 'health misinformation, fraud, and quackery'. This site provides information on a range of topics such as faith healing and psychic surgery as well as the more mainstream CAM treatments. It also produces a very readable e-mail consumer health newsletter. To subscribe to this news-letter send a blank e-mail (do not put anything in the subject line or the body of the text) to: <chdigest-subscribe@ssr.com>.

Conclusion

Before embarking upon an alternative therapy it is strongly advisable to discuss it first with your GP. Though the common perception is that alternative thera-pies are harmless – the worst they can do is do nothing – in reality this is not always the case. A recent issue of the *Annals of Internal Medicine* <http://www.annals.org/issues/v133n11/nts/200012050-00006.html> published a case report of a 55-year-old man with cancer of the sinus who died from kidney failure after taking hydrazine sulphate (a chemical used in rocket fuel). Advocates of hydrazine sulphate argue that it is effective in treating the progressive weight loss and body deterioration characteristic of advanced cancer. The man who died had been following the instructions provided on the Kathy Keeton Cancer Web site <http://www.kathykeeton-cancer.com/effective_therapy/page4.html>. Research into the use of this chemical shows that it provides no benefit to cancer patients <http://www.cancernet.nci.nih.gov/cam/hydrazine.htm>.

Discussion with your health professional will alert you to such issues and, if they believe that CAM may be worth trying, they may be able to recommend a particular practitioner. The finding that 40% of GPs have referred patients to a CAM practitioner shows how many health professionals are open to the idea that, for certain conditions, an alternative approach is worth considering. If your GP is unable to recommend a specific practitioner, the directory services described here may be useful.

As more information about CAM is published on the Internet we can be sure that the debate about its efficacy will continue. Let us hope, however, that the Internet will enable all of us to engage in this debate in a more informed way.

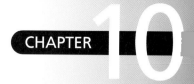

CHAPTER 10

Pregnancy, childbirth and infant care – information sources on the Internet

Introduction

For many women their first prolonged encounter with the health service starts when they become pregnant. Visits to the antenatal clinic, followed by a (hopefully) short stay in the maternity unit, and then home to care for the new infant are all life-changing events, and ones where the need for accurate and up-to-date information and advice becomes all too apparent. Is an amniocentesis test safe, will painkillers taken during labour harm the baby, and do the benefits of immunisation outweigh the dangers? These are a few of the many questions to which prospective parents want answers.

As with the other topics discussed in this book, we repeat the advice that your healthcare professional is the best person to answer these questions. That said, you might wish to find information in advance of a consultation, or do some follow-up research. In such cases the Internet is the obvious source to search.

In this chapter we highlight a number of high-quality Internet sources which prospective parents may find useful. With so much information available we have structured this chapter into three key sections – pregnancy, childbirth and infant care. It should be made clear, however, that most of the resources identified here will provide information on all aspects of pregnancy and childcare. The chapter concludes with a look at a number of pregnancy-related interactive tools and services.

Pregnancy

On becoming pregnant many women develop an almost insatiable thirst for information – a need the publishing industry has responded to with enthusiasm. Indeed, a visit to any bookshop will reveal a wealth of titles, covering all aspects of pregnancy. Books, however, represent just one part of the information chain. Magazines are another key information source and titles such as *Practical Parenting*, *Mother and Baby* and *Baby Magazine* are all readily available in the UK.

Into this crowded marketplace of information we now add the Internet. Here, information ranging from evidence-based studies on the best way to care for mother and baby, through to online tools that can be used to help parents choose a name for their new baby, is all readily available. The resources described here represent a taster of what is accessible via this electronic medium. If a specific subject you are interested in is not covered here – exercise in pregnancy, water births etc – please refer to Chapter 4 for help and advice on how to search the Internet.

Pregnancy – general resources

For an introductory overview of Internet resources relating to pregnancy, both the MEDLINE*plus* <http://www.medlineplus.gov> and the NHSDirect <http://www.nhsdirect.nhs.uk> services (discussed in Chapter 5) are highly recommended. The NHS Direct site, for example, provides information (and links to related resources) on topics such as planning a pregnancy and home birth as well as more health-focused issues including ectopic pregnancy and pre-eclampsia.

By design, these general health gateway services point to a relatively small number of resources. For a more comprehensive overview of the key health issues that arise during pregnancy the Obgyn.net <http://www.obgyn.net/pb/pb.asp> and the National Childbirth Trust (NCT) <http://www.nct-online.org> Web sites are worth exploring.

Obgyn.net – 'a global, physician reviewed network, for doctors, women and the medical industry' – provides access to a range of articles (written for a lay audience) on all aspects of pregnancy. Some of these articles include audio and video files. The site also includes a very active online forum <http://forums.obgyn.net/pregnancy-birth/> where women (and men) can post questions about pregnancy. What makes this forum particularly useful, is the fact that healthcare professionals who form part of the Obgyn.net editorial team respond to many of these queries (Fig. 10.1).

The Web site of the NCT <http://www.nct-online.org> has a number of online leaflets that provide information on topics such as alcohol and pregnancy, Caesarean section and home birth. For each topic the emphasis is on providing accurate, evidence-based information to help give every parent the opportunity to make an informed choice. The site also includes a practical guide to identifying reliable information – the advice is to view research critically – and provides the facility for new and prospective parents to order maternity items online from NCT Maternity Sales.

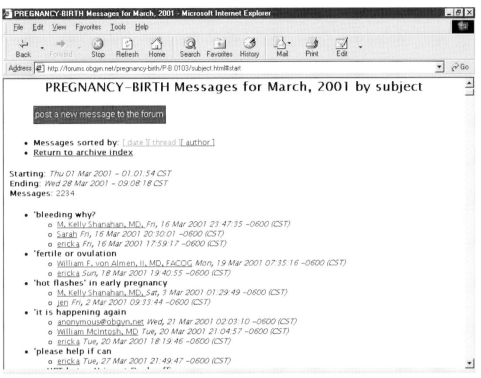

Fig. 10.1   Online discussion forum at Obgyn.net

Finally, in this section we draw attention to the Web site of the Maternity Alliance <http://www.maternityalliance.org.uk/>. One concern of many women have on learning they are pregnant pertains to their employment rights. The Maternity Alliance champions women's rights in this area and via its Web site it is possible to determine the current legislative position with regard to such issues as working whilst pregnant, maternity pay and parental leave.

Prenatal care

The MEDLINE*plus* site has pulled together a collection of Web-based resources that focus on prenatal care. Though the resources identified are US in origin, information about the need to stay healthy during pregnancy <http://www.kidshealth.org/parent/pregnancy_newborn/pregnancy/ preg_health.html> or the benefits of taking folic acid <http://www.cdc.gov/ nceh/cddh/fact/folnow.htm> are universal in nature.

As the pregnancy progresses it is natural to want to know what is happening to the developing baby and to the mother's body. For information on these subjects the Web site at Loyola University (Chicago) is particularly good

<http://www.luhs.org/health/topics/pregnant/index.htm>. Dividing the term of pregnancy into trimesters, information is given as to the likely size of the baby, how it is developing physically and mentally, and what changes the mother's body is having to make. It also provides a list of common symptoms (leg cramps, swelling of the ankles etc) that women may experience.

Tests and scans

During the course of a pregnancy the expectant mother may undergo various tests to determine whether the unborn baby is at risk from hereditary birth defects.

Information on both the maternal serum alpha fetoprotein test (MSAFP) and the triple test has been produced by the Mayo Clinic <http://www.mayoclinic.com/home?id=PR00015>. Both of these online leaflets use a question and answer format and address concerns such as what the tests are for, how they are done and what the results mean.

These tests may in turn indicate that further tests – such as amniocentesis and chorionic villus sampling (CVS) – should be performed. The March of Dimes Birth Defect Foundation Web site provides information about these in a clear and comprehensible style that spells out the relative risk each one poses to the unborn child. Details of the amniocentesis and the CVS tests are available at <http://www.modimes.org/HealthLibrary2/factsheets/amniocentesis.htm> and <http://www.modimes.org/HealthLibrary2/FactSheets/Chorionic_villus_sampling.htm>.

The expectant mother may also have a number of ultrasound scans. These scans are used to answer a range of questions, such as how the baby is developing, or to rule out or confirm a suspected ectopic pregnancy. For comprehensive information about ultrasound in pregnancy the Web site created by obstetrician Dr Joseph Woo is a 'must-see' <http://www.ob-ultrasound.net/>. This site provides information about when and why ultrasound is used, what the safety issues are, and describes the various types of ultrasound procedures (including 3-D ultrasound). It also has a significant collection of online images and videos that detail a baby's development from seven weeks (Fig. 10.2).

Miscarriage and stillbirth

Not every pregnancy ends happily and when a miscarriage or stillbirth occurs the need for information – why this has happened, who I can talk to, what I do next – may be considerable.

In the UK, the Miscarriage Association <http://www.the-ma.org.uk/> has produced a number of information leaflets on miscarriage, including one that provides help and advice to people who know someone who has suffered a

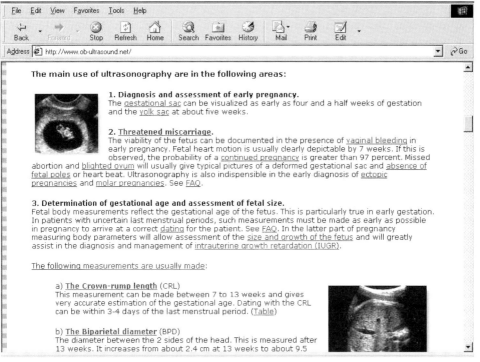

Fig. 10.2   Ultrasound scans – Joseph Woo's ultrasound site

miscarriage. Advice given here includes the need to acknowledge the baby and provides tips on what not to say.

The Stillbirth and Neonatal Deaths Society (SANDS) provides support for bereaved parents (and their families) whose baby has died at or soon after birth. The Web site <http://www.uk-sands.org/> gives details of how to find a local support group.

Childbirth

As the big day approaches the information needs of the pregnant woman become more focused on the actual process of giving birth and how best to care for her newborn infant. This section will highlight Web resources that address these needs.

Childbirth – general resources

Many of the sites discussed thus far in this chapter provide information on issues relating to childbirth. One additional resource that may be of interest is the Pregnancy and Birth Web site <http://www.childbirth.org>. Run by a group of parents, nurses and midwives this site promotes the view that 'birth is a natural process – not a medical procedure'. As well as providing a number of fact-sheets on a range of childbirth-related topics, the site also hosts a lively chat room and provides links to further resources.

Giving birth

One common concern many women experience pertains to the amount of pain relief they may require during labour and the possible adverse effect this may have on the baby. In recognition of this the American Association of Nurse Anesthetists <http://www.aana.com/patients/options.asp> have produced a patient-friendly guide, outlining the anaesthetic options available during labour. Though it makes sense for the expectant mother to discuss the pain relief options with her midwife, this document may help inform that process.

For many women a Caesarean section will be required to deliver the baby. Indeed, one in every six pregnant women in the UK has a Caesarean section. The NCT is concerned by this trend and on its Web site it demands that women are given balanced information about the relative benefits, risks and alternatives <http://www.nct-online.org/caesarean2.htm>.

For information on the actual Caesarean section procedure – complete with detailed line drawings and clinical images – the YourSurgery.com Web site <http://www.yoursurgery.com/data/Procedures/c_section/p_c_section.htm> is worth a visit.

Finally, information about what to do when the due date has passed <http://familydoctor.org/handouts/143.html>, and what steps can be taken to induce labour <http://familydoctor.org/handouts/450.html>, has been produced by the American Academy of Family Physicians. Obviously, if these eventualities come to pass the expectant mother will be in close contact with her healthcare team. However, being alert to these possibilities and aware of what actions can be taken, may help to reduce the inevitable anxieties.

Infant care

The arrival of a new baby is invariably a time of great joy and worry. After nine months of waiting, parents are suddenly presented with a new child that demands almost continuous 24-hour care. For first-time parents this workload is exacerbated by the usual fear that they do not really know what they are doing. As well as these fairly natural concerns there are also questions that need to be answered and decisions that have to be taken. Will formula feed have an adverse effect on the baby's development? Should the baby be immunised? What are the risks and benefits to the newborn infant from a vitamin K jab?

As has been stressed previously, such questions should be discussed with your healthcare team. That said, there will be times when you seek additional information, not least so you understand the options and the consequences of your decisions.

Infant care – general resources

The NCT have produced a wealth of high-quality information on how best to care for the child, much of which is available online through the 'Life with a new baby' Web pages <http://www.nct-online.org/lifewithnewbaby.htm>. Issues covered here include a series of tips on how you can enjoy the first few weeks with your child (despite being exhausted), how to cope with colic, and a guide to some of the reflexes the newborn baby will exhibit.

For a more comprehensive information source about infant care the Kidshealth.org site <http://kidshealth.org/parent/pregnancy_newborn/index.html> is highly respected. Here, information is categorised into various discrete sections, such as 'Common conditions', 'Communicating with your

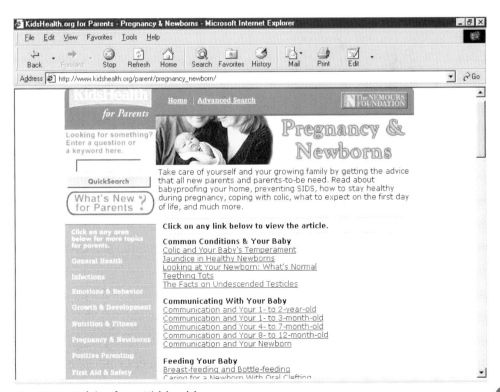

Fig. 10.3   Advice from Kidshealth.org

baby', and 'Playing with your baby' (Fig. 10.3). The site also has a section on 'Home and family issues' that gives guidance on how to baby-proof your home, and preparing your child for a new sibling. The kidshealth site is produced by the Nemours Foundation, a non-profit organisation devoted to children's health.

Feeding

The MEDLINE*plus* directory has an excellent collection of links to Internet resources that provide information and advice on infant feeding <http://www.nlm.nih.gov/medlineplus/breastfeeding.html>. Many of these sites focus on breast-feeding (and the benefits that both mother and baby derive from it) and its practical implications, such as how to prevent sore nipples <http://www.aafp.org/fpr/980300fr/23.html> and how to use a breast pump <http://www.mayoclinic.com/home?id=PR00002>.

Not every mother, however, is able or willing to breast-feed and in such cases information about formula feeding may be sought. One source that addresses this need is the ParentsPlace Web site <http://www.parentsplace.com/expert/nutritionist/bottlefeeding/>. Here, nutritionists provide advice on a range of questions such as 'Can a new-born be overfed?' and 'Does iron in formula cause constipation?' in a non-judgmental and supportive manner. As the baby develops, other sections of this site will prove useful such as 'Feeding your toddler' <http://www.parentsplace.com/expert/nutritionist/foodjuice/> and 'Dealing with picky eaters' <http://www.parentsplace.com/expert/nutritionist/picky/>.

Immunisation, vaccination and childhood diseases

Consenting to give your healthy child any injection is invariably difficult. Such difficulties are exacerbated when there is a debate raging between respected professionals over the relative safety of a particular vaccine, as recently witnessed in the UK over the MMR (measles, mumps, rubella) vaccine.

Faced with real-life dilemmas – should my child have the MMR vaccine and be protected from these diseases or are the perceived risks too great? – it is inevitable (and desirable) that parents will turn to the Internet to find more information about childhood immunisation.

Health Promotion England (the successor to the Health Education Authority) have recently launched the 'Childhood immunisation and vaccination' Web site <http://www.immunisation.org.uk/>. This site aims to provide parents with 'accurate, up-to-date and fully researched information on childhood, pre-school and school (adolescent) immunisations'. In addition to providing clearly written patient guides on all of the core childhood vaccinations, the site also includes a ready reference guide to when these vaccinations should be administered and how.

In the US the Center for Disease Control provides similar information, though via the 'ABC's of safe and healthy child care' <http://www.cdc.gov/ncidod/hip/abc/facts.htm> you can also find fact-sheets on a number of other childhood diseases, such as chickenpox and influenza.

Interactive tools

Thus far this chapter has focused on the role the Internet can play in helping parents make informed decisions about the care of their baby. In addition to this the Internet also provides access to a range of interactive tools and services that new and prospective parents may find useful.

Ovulation calculator

There are a number of online ovulation calculators that women can use to help determine when they are more likely to conceive. One of the more

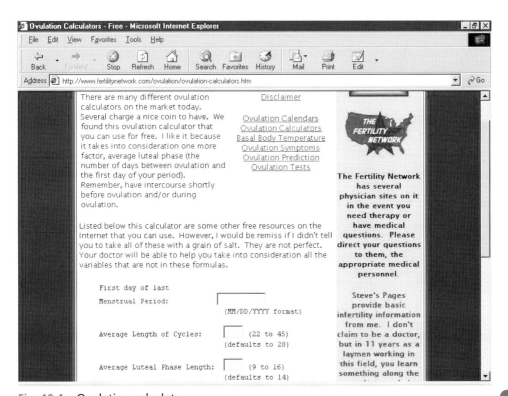

Fig. 10.4   Ovulation calculator

sophisticated calculators has been produced by the Infertility Network <http://www.infertilitynetwork.com/ovulation/ovulation-calculators.htm>. Based on three variables – the first day of the last menstrual period, the average length of the cycles, and the average luteal phase – this calculator will estimate the next ovulation date, and (assuming that the woman becomes pregnant) provide an approximate due date (Fig. 10.4). The Parenthood Web site <http://www.parenthoodweb.com/parent_cfmfiles/PregOvulate.cfm> provides a similar service, though this allows you to see an estimated ovulation date over a 12-month period.

Birth plans

Birth plans are a simple and non-confrontational way for pregnant women to inform the healthcare team about their personal preferences with regard to the delivery of their baby. Typically, creating a comprehensive birth plan has been a somewhat confusing and time-consuming process. The development of online birth plans, however, has simplified this task.

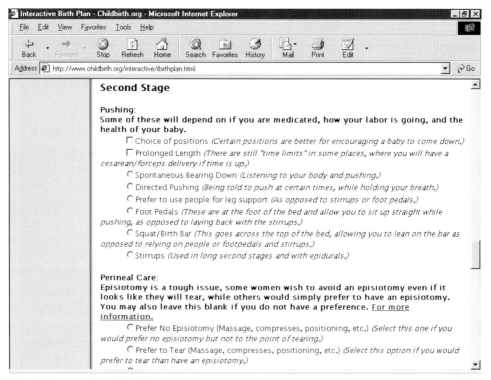

Fig. 10.5   Online birth plan

At the Childbirth.org site <**http://www.childbirth.org/interactive/ibirthplan.html**> expectant mothers can draw up a detailed plan that can be printed and taken to the maternity hospital (Fig.10.5). The plan covers topics such as the preferred level of pain relief and the desired position when giving birth. The form has some in-built verification features that will not allow you to choose two mutually exclusive things. For example, you cannot have continuous monitoring with a fetoscope, nor can you breast-feed only with a bottle.

Choosing a name

Choosing a name for the new baby is a game prospective parents (and their friends) play with relish. And, though the Internet will not be able to resolve the inevitable disputes that arise over the choice of the name, the baby-name finder pages <**http://www.parentsplace.com/pregnancy/babynames/finder/**> will almost certainly come up with additional names you had never thought of. Figure 10.6 shows how you can search for a name based on the number of syllables you desire, the starting letter and the language.

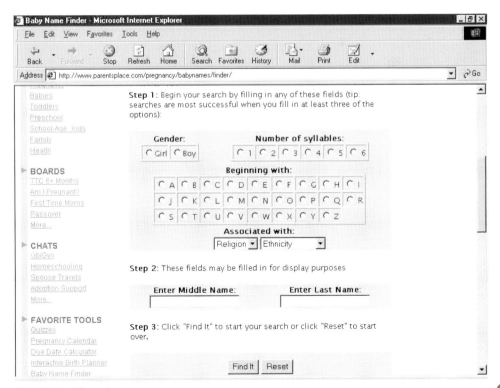

Fig. 10.6   Choosing a name

The 'Mystic Baby Namer' <http://www.childbirth.org/interactive/babynamer.html> program uses a single character trait (sassy, carefree, independent etc.) to select a name. This service should not be taken seriously!

In a similar vein you may wish to determine the sex of the unborn baby. At the 'Is it a boy or girl interactive test' <http://www.childbirth.org/articles/boyorgirl.html> site this can be done without recourse to ultrasound scans etc. Instead, this information is derived from a series of old wives' tales. For example, if the abdomen looks like a watermelon it must be a girl, if it looks like a basketball it must be a boy. Again not to be taken seriously, but what this site lacks in evidence it makes up for in entertainment!

Conclusion

In its 'Top 10 tips for labour' <http://www.nct-online.org/10TopTipsForLabour.htm> the NCT emphasises the importance of being informed. Though the suggested routes for this are antenatal classes, books and videos, as this chapter has demonstrated the Internet can be another excellent source for information on all aspects of pregnancy and childcare.

Keeping safe

Overview

Throughout this book attention has been paid to the quality of health information available on the Internet. As the Internet enables *anyone* to publish *anything* we need to adopt a healthy scepticism towards the information we find.

Chapter 11 looks at the issue of quality and highlights the different types of misinformation perpetrated on the Internet. These include 'cure-all' remedies – where a single alternative therapy is presented as a magic bullet solution – and lifestyle scams which, for example, offer a simple, painless way to lose weight, counter baldness, and improve one's sexual performance.

Critical evaluation of the information we find on the Internet is the best way to protect ourselves from this type of information. In recognition of this, this chapter also introduces the concept of critical appraisal and highlights a number of online tools that can be used to help develop these skills.

Chapter 12 brings together many of the themes covered in this book and considers to what extent the Internet has led to the rise of the empowered patient. This chapter includes information on how best to prepare for the doctor/patient consultation and discusses the most effective ways of presenting the information you have found on the Internet to your doctor.

The final chapter looks to the future and the possible role the Internet will play in the delivery of health care.

CHAPTER 11

Quality of health information on the Internet

Introduction

The quality of health information on the Internet is extremely variable. On searching for, say, 'cancer' using the more general Internet search tools like AltaVista or Google (see Chapter 4), one can move seamlessly from authoritative sites like Cancernet <http://www.nci.nih.gov> and OncoLink <http://cancer.med.upenn.edu>, through to highly dubious ones such as the 'Cancer can now be cured' site. Run by Hulda Clark, an 'independent research scientist', visitors to this site are informed that:

All cancers are alike. They are all caused by a parasite ... and if you kill the parasite, the cancer stops immediately.

The site goes on to explain that these parasites can be removed – 'safely and without any side effects' – by a low-voltage device, known as a Syncrometer Zapper.

Though it would be nice to believe that one of the biggest killers in the Western world could be defeated by a simple 'zap', there is, unfortunately, no evidence of any kind that this treatment has any effect on any form of cancer. Moreover, though in itself the Zapper will do little harm – independent tests reveal that it is little more than a galvanometer that measures skin resistance – there is a real danger that some patients will try this method *before* seeking appropriate care and treatment. This delay may be fatal.

Misinformation of the kind perpetrated by Hulda Clark is not the only problem that besets the consumer. Web sites that are highly biased and present only one side of the argument are another concern, as is the facility to buy drugs and medical devices that may be unregulated, unproven and potentially dangerous.

In this chapter we provide examples of these types of sites, discuss what attempts are being made to regulate health information on the Internet and, most importantly, provide practical guidelines that will help you to appraise the quality of the information you find.

Misinformation on the Web

Although examples of medical misinformation on the Internet are numerous, analysis shows that they all fit within one of the following distinct groups:

- **'Cure-all' remedies**
  Here a single alternative therapy is presented as a 'magic bullet' solution.
- **Lifestyle scams**
  Sites in this category typically offer a painless way to lose weight, improve sexual performance etc.
- **Evidence by anecdote**
  Personal experiences are presented as facts – no reference is made to any independently published research.
- **Biased information**
  Only one side of the argument is presented to the reader.
- **Dangerous devices**
  Sites in this category typically try to sell the unwary consumer a medical device that should only be used by a qualified professional.

We look in turn at each of these categories, highlighting specific sites that promote these forms of misinformation.

Cure-all remedies

It should come as no surprise to learn that unscrupulous marketeers use the Internet to peddle various miracle cures. The cost of setting up a credible-looking Web site is negligible, whilst the potential profits are huge. Typically, these sites target those people with chronic medical conditions for which there are no known cures.

Cancer patients are an obvious target and one cure-all treatment that has received a lot of attention over the past couple of years is laetrile (also known as amygdalin or 'vitamin B17'), a concoction made of apricot seeds. For example, at the Cure4Cancer site <http://www.1cure4cancer.com/> visitors are informed that '7 to 10 apricot seeds per day will make it impossible to develop cancer in one's life time'. If you already have cancer you are advised to start eating apricot seeds, safe in the knowledge that 'most of the people that already have cancer clusters in their body, who eat the apricot seeds and/or take the vitamin B17 show near to complete tumor regression' (Fig.11.1).

What this site fails to disclose are the results of clinical trials that have taken

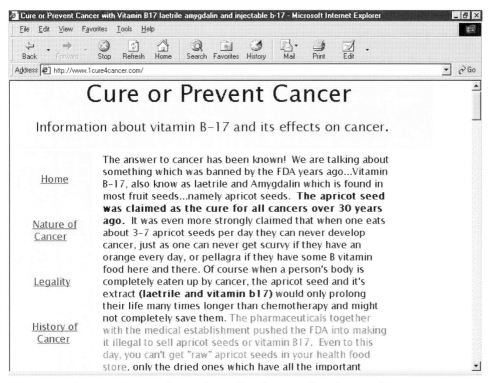

Fig. 11.1   The Cure4Cancer site – advocating the use of apricot seeds

place into laetrile. These show that laetrile has no anticancer activity in humans, and that the side effects of this 'therapy' mirror the symptoms of cyanide poisoning. [For further details see <http://cancernet.nci.nih.gov/cam/ laetrile.htm>.]

Hydrazine sulphate is another unproven cancer treatment which is actively promoted by numerous Web sites. For example, the KathyKeeton Web site <http://www.kathykeeton-cancer.com/> states that:

Hydrazine sulfate has been used by thousands of desperate cancer patients over the past 25 years with remarkable results. Although it has in many cases caused complete remission of cancer, hydrazine sulfate is primarily an anti-cachexia drug. Studies performed in the former U.S.S.R. and UCLA Medical Center demonstrate improvements in appetite, weight gain, albumin maintenance (albumin is a blood protein and low levels of it are an extremely accurate predictor of mortality), energy levels, quality of life and, in terminal patients, survival time. It also appears to have ameliorating effects when taken during chemotherapy, and especially with radiation therapy.

In contrast, the US National Cancer Institute reports that studies into hydrazine sulphate have shown:

> *Hydrazine sulfate has shown no antitumor activity in randomised clinical trials and data concerning its effectiveness in treating cancer-related cachexia are inconclusive*
> <http://cancernet.nci.nih.gov/cam/hydrazine.htm>.

Even more disturbing is the recent article in the medical journal the *Annals of Internal Medicine*, which reported on a 55-year-old man who died from kidney failure after taking hydrazine sulfate <http://www.annals.org/issues/v133n11/nts/200012050-00006.html>.

Though cancer patients seem to be the main target for this type of misinformation, they are not alone. Arthritis sufferers are also offered a number of 'miracle cures'. The Vital Force Web site <http://www.vital-force.net/>, for example, offers cis-9-cetylmyristoleate (CMO) capsules as a quick, painless cure:

> *Arthritis pain can be reduced by nearly 70–100% in almost every instance. Inflammation can be reduced by nearly 70–100% in almost every case. Although nothing works 100% of the time for 100% of the people, studies show that CMO has a very high success rate.*

Where these studies were published is not disclosed. A search of the MEDLINE database, however, fails to find *any* information about the effectiveness of this nutritional supplement in managing arthritis.

Lifestyle scams

Medical quackery is a business that sells false hope. Not all of this business, however, is aimed at the chronically ill. Many sites prey on the wishful thinking of those who seek shortcuts to weight loss and improvements in their personal appearance and performance.

Good examples of this are the Web sites that sell so-called slimming soaps. At the Warmlife.com site <http://www.warmlife.com/cellulite%20soap.htm>, potential customers are encouraged to 'lather up and watch your pounds melt off' (Fig. 11.2).

Another site selling this soap <http://www.demandby.com/seaweedeng.htm> provides the following user-instructions:

> 1. *Use as normal bath soap but lather and massage into the body areas where you would require slimming approximately a minute. Do not leave on body parts that do not require slimming like your breast for more than a minute as it will slim those parts of your body.*
>
> 2. *Massage and lather into your body parts that require slimming about 40*

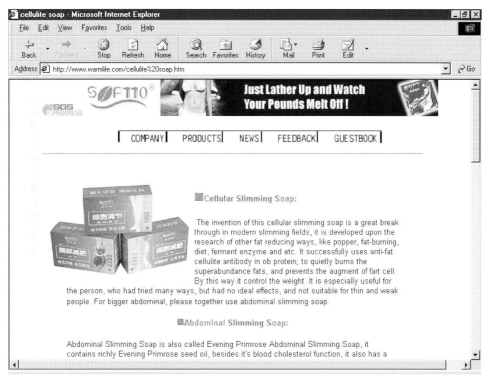

Fig. 11.2   Slimming soap – 'lather up and watch the pounds melt off'

> *times or about a minute. Areas that can be effectively trim down is your huge tummy, big thigh and large legs* [sic].

People seeking information about hair loss are another group who may stumble across Web sites with outlandish claims. The Sheng Chi Regenerative Herbal Shampoo <http://www.4rhythm.com/sham.html> has properties that (allegedly) 'promote re-growth of lost hair for all hair types male and female'. To get the maximum benefit the site suggests that you use a minimum of 6 bottles. Each bottle retails at US$8.00.

Finally, anyone seeking information about impotence (or related sexual problems) needs to be alert to the numerous Web sites that promise to 'improve your sexual performance'. Following the licensing of Viagra, numerous herbal alternatives appeared on the Web. For example, at the Viagra Alternatives site <http://www.viagraalternatives.net> consumers can choose from a range of natural products such as 'Herbal Rise' and 'X-treme V'. The latter is described as 'a super potent sexual enhancement formula for men', that 'requires no prescription, is safe and effective'.

Precisely what this product does is outside our scope. However, the small print disclaimer at the foot of the Web page probably tells us all we need to know:

> *The statements regarding this product have not been evaluated by the Food and Drug Administration. This product is not intended to diagnose, treat, cure or prevent any disease.*

With this sort of testimony it is difficult to believe that this product does anything at all!

Evidence by anecdote

Not all medical misinformation on the Web has a commercial agenda. There are numerous Web sites where individual users and organisations post information in good faith, oblivious of the fact that it is inaccurate or misleading.

A study published in the *British Medical Journal* examining the quality of information on the Web that pertained to managing a child with fever, concluded that only 10% of sites adhered closely to published recommendations. Some sites advocated treatments such as cold sponging, or sponging with alcohol – both of which are potentially dangerous. [Details of this study can be found at: <http://www.bmj.com/cgi/content/full/314/7098/1875>.]

Perhaps even more worrying were the results of another study, published in the journal *Pediatrics*. This found that 80% of pages authored by medical institutions, schools and hospitals that discussed the management of childhood diarrhoea, did *not* conform with best practices as defined by the American Academy of Paediatricians. [Details of this study can be found at: <http://www.pediatrics.org/cgi/content/full/101/6/e2>.]

Misinformation, however, is not restricted to Web sites. One other study that considered the information posted to the Internet newsgroup *sci.med. pharmacy* <news://sci.med.pharmacy> concluded that around 20% of all postings were potentially harmful. [See: <http://www.ncbi.nlm.nih.gov/entrez/query.fcgi?cmd=Retrieve&db=PubMed&list_uids=9519647&dopt=Abstract>.]

What these studies serve to show is that information based on personal testimonies – that make little or no reference to any supporting published research – should be treated with great caution.

Biased information

The Web provides a vehicle for every pressure group to promote their views and beliefs to a world-wide audience. Consequently, another issue to which consumers need to be alert is biased information.

In some cases this may be easy to spot (and to avoid). Anyone looking for information on, say, the effectiveness of the morning-after pill (mifepristone) can probably deduce that they are unlikely to find an objective and balanced view at the Web sites of pro-life organisations, such as the American Life League <http://www.all.org/> or Abortion is Murder <http://abortionismurder.org/>.

In some cases, however, bias can be far more subtle and harder to detect. For example, at the official-sounding National Vaccine Information Center <http://www.909shot.com> visitors are informed of a thriving two-month-old baby who died after being given the diphtheria-pertussis-tetanus vaccine (DPT), and the death of a 13-day-old baby following a hepatatitis B injection.

This site is not part of a government-sponsored campaign to alert parents to the potential dangers of childhood immunisation, but a national non-profit educational organisation, founded by parents whose children were injured or died following vaccine reactions. Not surprisingly, therefore, the site presents a fairly one-sided and negative view of childhood vaccination.

Though it is important that such concerns are publicised and brought to the attention of parents, there is a need to balance this information with the positive benefits of childhood immunisation.

Dangerous devices

One other area of concern is the relative ease by which patients can buy DIY health devices on the Internet. In June 1997 the US Food and Drug Administration published a warning to consumers that home abortion kits (available via the Internet) posed 'significant, possibly life threatening health risks'. A subsequent health hazard assessment concluded that the use of this kit without a physician's supervision could 'cause heavy vaginal bleeding and even death'.

Human Immunodeficiency Virus (HIV) testing kits are another concern – due mainly to the fact that the results they provide are highly unreliable. Consequently, in the case of a false negative result, there is a real danger that people who have this virus will delay seeking appropriate care, believing that the results of their home test were accurate. Despite the fact that in the UK it is an offence under the HIV Testing Kits and Service Regulations to sell such kits, there are numerous Web sites promoting and selling this product to consumers throughout the world.

Quality initiatives

In an attempt to protect consumers from the types of information (and products) discussed here, a number of organisations have developed mechanisms to evaluate Web sites and give 'badges of approval' to those that meet a defined quality threshold.

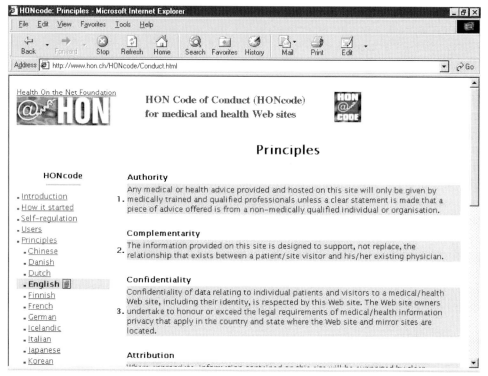

Fig. 11.3   Health on the Net (HON) logo – a sign of quality

One of the more successful schemes has been developed by the Geneva-based Health on the Net Foundation (HON). Here, Web sites that comply with an eight-point Code of Conduct are granted the right to display the Health on the Net logo on their pages. This internationally recognised stamp of quality is analogous to the British Standard kite-mark (Fig. 11.3).

Central to this Code is the principle that any medical information must 'only be given by medically trained and qualified professionals'. Where this condition cannot be met there must be a 'clear statement that a piece of advice offered is from a non-medically qualified individual or organisation'. Full details of the Code can be found at: <http://www.hon.ch/HONcode/Conduct.html>.

Concerns that the HON logo can be copied – and applied to any Web site – has prompted the development of a number of more sophisticated schemes. The Health Internet Ethics consortium (which includes some of the biggest US consumer sites such as drKoop.com and InteliHealth) are developing an E-Health seal. Here, sites that comply with the 14 principles developed by the consortium – relating to privacy, quality, accountability etc – will be able to display this seal. The seal, however, will be dynamic and by clicking on it visitors will be taken to the independent TRUSTe site where details of the site display-ing the seal can be verified. Details of the principles developed by the Health Internet Ethics consortium are available at: <http://www.hiethics.org/Principles/index.asp>.

A similar scheme, MedCERTAIN, <http://www.medcertain.org/> is currently being funded by the EU. Unlike the HiEthics scheme, MedCERTAIN will be a decentralised system whereby qualified individuals and organisations will rank Web sites. This ranking will span from simple quality seals indicating a 'good standing' of the site to 'gold' quality seals indicating that the site has been independently peer-reviewed.

Undoubtedly, the development of these badges and seals is of great use to the consumer. If you happen to come across a site that displays one of these badges you can be assured that the information will be of a reasonably high quality.

However, we do not believe that badging systems will ever provide all the solutions to the quality issue. There are simply too many health sites to badge – and if we took the simplistic view that you should only use those sites that have been badged you will exclude the majority of health Web sites. To put this in context, sites such as the National Cancer Institute, NHSDirect or the BMJ – all of which provide high-quality information – would have to be ignored as none of these display any 'quality assured' badge.

A more realistic solution is to encourage health consumers to appraise critically and evaluate carefully the information they find on the Internet.

Evaluating medical information

Critical appraisal is something most of us do all the time, albeit unconsciously. Thus, a news item broadcast by the BBC might be believed, whereas a story in a tabloid newspaper might be treated with more caution.

On the Internet, however, where many of the sites are new and have not yet been able to build up a reputation for providing high quality information, the appraisal process is more difficult. Put simply, how can users looking for information on, say, psoriasis, differentiate between the National Psoriasis Foundation site <http://www.psoriasis.org> and the Psoriasis Treatment site <http://www.psoriasis.com>?

One relatively simple way to evaluate information on the Internet is to use the four-point checklist developed by Silberg and the American Medical Association (Box 11.1). Sites that fail to comply with these minimum standards should be rejected.

These criteria, however, do not address the equally important issues of whether the information is appropriate, or presented in a way that the con-sumer can readily understand. In recognition of these issues – and others – a

Box 11.1　Evaluating Web pages – Silberg criteria

- **Authorship**

  The author(s) of a Web page, along with their affiliations and credentials, should be clearly stated.
- **Attribution**

  If a Web site is citing research or evidence then the source of this data must be explicitly stated. Ideally, there should be a hypertext link to the original research.
- **Disclosure**

  The owner of the Web site must be prominently displayed, along with any sponsorship or advertising deals that could constitute a potential conflict of interest.
- **Currency**

  Web pages should indicate when they were first created and last updated.

Based on the recommendations developed by Silberg WM, Lundberg GD, Musacchio RA. Assessing, controlling, and assuring the quality of medical information on the Internet: caveant lector et viewor – let the reader and viewer beware. JAMA. 1997;277:1244–1245.

number of rating tools have been developed to help users develop critical appraisal skills. The most significant of these are the DISCERN Instrument <http://www.discern.org.uk> and Health Information Technology Institute (HITI) IQ Tool <http://hitiweb.mitretek.org/iq/>. Using these tools anyone can critically appraise any Web site.

DISCERN

DISCERN is a brief questionnaire that provides users with a 'valid and reliable way of assessing the quality of written information on treatment choices for a health problem'.

Based on 15 questions, the DISCERN Instrument encourages consumers to think about issues such as whether the information is balanced and unbiased and whether or not areas of uncertainty are properly explained. Beyond these core quality issues the Instrument also examines the quality of information as it pertains to treatment choices. For example, though a site may score well in that it provides evidence-based information, it may score poorly on issues such as explaining how a treatment works, or by *not* describing what would happen

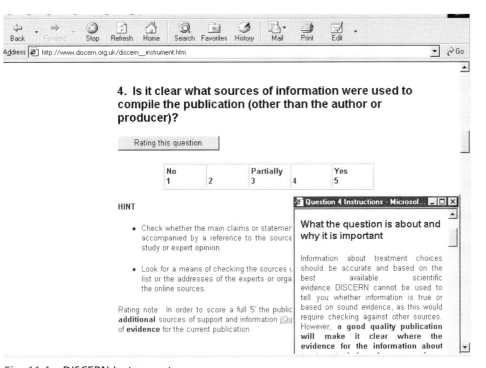

Fig. 11.4 DISCERN Instrument

if no treatment were administered. Only when all the questions posed by DISCERN have been answered can a decision be made as to whether the site contains useful and appropriate information.

Figure 11.4 shows some of the questions in the Instrument. Each question is accompanied by a series of tips and hints to help guide and educate the user.

IQ Tool

Similar to DISCERN, the IQ Tool provides another checklist of questions consumers should ask when visiting any medical Web site. Unlike DISCERN, the IQ Tool actually calculates a final quality score, based on the answers you provide. It is important to remember, however, that this score is a reflection of how well a site answered the questions. It is no guarantee that a site is either good or bad. Having said that, each report provides detailed information on what was missing from the site and why these omissions are important. Figures 11.5 and 11.6 show a selection of the questions asked by the IQ Tool and an example of a scored report.

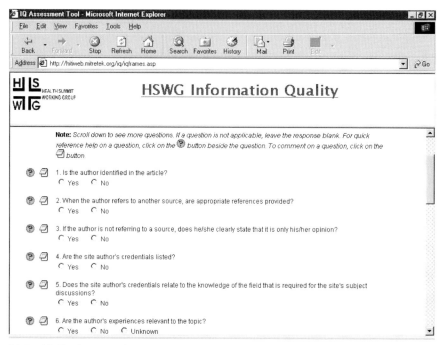

Fig. 11.5   IQ Tool – questions

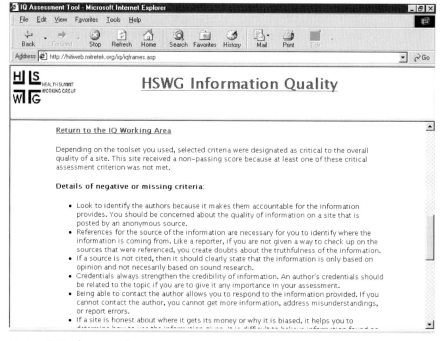

Fig. 11.6   IQ Tool – scored report

Conclusion

As anyone can set up a Web site and publish whatever they like, or post any message to Internet discussion lists and newsgroups, all Internet users need to be alert to the dangers of misleading and inaccurate information. As discussed above, in some cases inaccurate medical information can be fatal.

Using the tools, techniques and services discussed in this chapter, however, consumers can develop the necessary critical appraisal skills. With these skills all Web sites can be evaluated and the true potential of the Internet can be realised.

The empowered patient?

Introduction

In a listlessness of despair I turned over the pages. I came to typhoid fever – read the symptoms – discovered that I had typhoid fever, must have had it for months without knowing it – wondered what else I had got; turned up St Vitus's dance – found as I expected that I had that too. Cholera I had with severe complications; and diptheria I seem to have been born with. I plodded through the 26 letters, and the only malady I could conclude I had not got was housemaid's knee.

I walked into that reading room a happy healthy man. I walked out a decrepit wreck.

So spoke the hapless 'J' in Jerome K Jerome's *Three Men in a Boat,* after consulting a medical dictionary. On seeking help for his condition, J's doctor wrote out a prescription that concluded with the advice, 'don't stuff your head with things you don't understand'.

Though Jerome's novel was written over 100 years ago, the advice given could have been written more recently with patients seeking medical information on the Internet in mind. As if to prove the point, an article in *The Times* newspaper (10 February 2001) began:

The other week a GP told me, with both amusement and resignation, that his latest dread was the patient with the file. Not the patient's own file, you understand, but a file, often inches thick of medical diagnoses and treatments downloaded from the Internet. However, while it may be helpful for the patient to feel he is 'taking control' of his or her, often entirely misdiagnosed illness, those sheaves of paper bring nothing but difficulty for the doctor.

Consequently, if using the Internet turns us all into hypochondriacs (or cyber-chondriacs) and the information we give to the doctor presents nothing but difficulties, is there any value in using this medium – and the wealth of resources we have highlighted in this book – to become an informed patient?

Needless to say we believe there is. Perhaps what these two quotations serve to show is that the patient who goes to their doctor armed with a ready diagnosis and preferred course of treatment is unlikely to receive a warm welcome. As we have stressed elsewhere, finding information on the Internet does not turn us into diagnosticians and surgeons. Instead, the Internet provides a means by which we can become more informed about our health and as a consequence become a more equal partner in the doctor/patient relationship.

In many ways, however, this is easier said than done. Many people may feel very uncomfortable about appearing as an equal with their doctor. Specifically, many may worry about how their doctor will react if they present information which contradicts – or is at variance – with the treatment regime their doctor has recommended. Though the fear may be unfounded, the patient may also feel that they will be treated differently if they appear to be more informed than the professional.

In recognition of these very real concerns this chapter will highlight a number of ways in which the patient can present information to their doctor in an effective and non-threatening way. We will also highlight a number of Internet resources that can be used to help prepare the patient for the consultation, focusing in particular on those sites that provide a series of questions that the patient could/should ask.

Preparing for the consultation

For many people a visit to the doctor can be a daunting prospect. Will something serious be discovered? Is that test necessary? Is it routine, or does it indicate something far more serious? Is that medication addictive? Is surgery the only option? These are just a few of the many questions patients may want to ask, but through a combination of fear, embarrassment and confusion find they cannot.

One way such problems can be mitigated is to prepare a list of questions in advance of the consultation. Such a list will help you to focus on the key topics that need to be discussed and clarified, and by thinking of these issues in advance, the twin emotions of fear and embarrassment can be better managed.

In response to these common concerns a number of Web sites have published a series of questions (*aides-mémoire*) patients can refer to and use during the consultation. For example, the National Cancer Institute's *'Questions to ask your doctor about breast cancer'* advises patients to seek answers to a range of questions, including 'What tests will I have to have

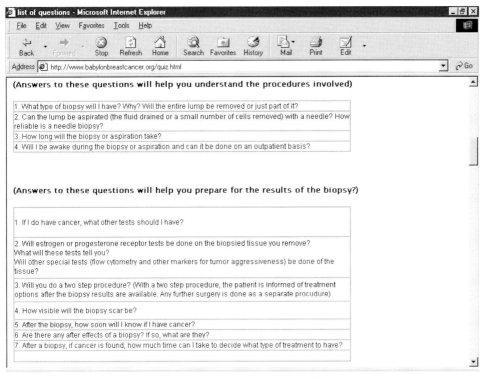

Fig. 12.1   National Cancer Institute – questions to ask about breast cancer

before surgery?', 'What are the treatment options?' and 'What are the risks and benefits of these procedures?' (Fig. 12.1).

Though these questions sound obvious – as indeed they are – they may not be easy to call to mind if you have just been told that you have breast cancer. Studies show that many patients who are told that they have cancer (any type) leave the consultation 'unsure about the diagnosis and prognosis, confused about the meaning of – and need for – further diagnostic tests, unclear about the management plan and uncertain about the true therapeutic intent of treatment'. [Fallowfield L, Jenkins V 'Effective communication skills are the key to good cancer care' *European Journal of Cancer*, 1999; 35(11):1592–1597 <http://www.ncbi.nlm.nih.gov/entrez/query.fcgi?cmd=Retrieve&db=PubMed &list_uids=10673967>]

In addition to providing advice on what questions to ask, many of these Web sites also provide practical help on how to manage the responses. Suggestions include taking a notepad and pen to record what you are told, and not accepting 'gobbledegook' or 'techno-babble'. If you do not understand something then tell your doctor and get them to explain it again. Every profession has its own jargon, which to an outsider can be meaningless. So, just as the authors of this book would not expect all doctors to be au fait with library-related concepts and jargon – AACR2, MARC21 and interoperability, to list but three – it is unreasonable to expect the health consumer to understand everything a health professional may tell them.

To help prepare for a consultation see the information presented in Tables 12.1 and 12.2. Table 12.1 identifies a number of Web sites that provide general advice on the type of questions to ask your doctor, whilst Table 12.2 looks at a number of sites that provide disease-specific questions.

Table 12.1   Asking the right questions

General questions
<http://www.pocketdoctor.co.uk/doctorq>

Devised by Dr Phil Hammond this site provides patients with a range of questions – pertaining to different scenarios – patients could ask their doctor. For example, if the doctor is unable to offer a diagnosis Dr Hammond recommends asking 'Are there any tests that would help make the diagnosis?' or 'What should I do if the symptoms don't go or get worse?'. Other areas covered include what to ask if you are considering complementary therapy or are offered a prescription medicine.

Questions to ask before surgery
<http://www.ahcpr.gov/consumer/surgery.htm>

Although television may have removed some of the mystique of the operating theatre, the prospect of surgery is always going to be frightening. Most operations, however, are not emergencies and this means you have time to ask your surgeon questions about the operation and decide whether or not to proceed.

The US Agency for Health Care Policy and Research (AHCPR) has compiled a series of questions you may wish to ask your surgeon. These include 'What are the benefits of having the operation?' and 'What are the risks?'. For each question, explanatory notes are provided which could act as additional question prompts (Fig. 12.2).

Questions to ask before a medical test
<http://cpmcnet.columbia.edu/texts/guide/hmg12_0002.html>

No one should have any medical test without being fully informed about what it entails and why the doctor is recommending it. To help the patient become more informed in this area, a team from the Columbia Presbyterian Medical Center have compiled a list of questions (with supporting notes) which patients should ask the doctor before undergoing a test. Suggested questions include 'How accurate is the test?', 'What might cause a false positive or false negative or other inaccurate result?', 'What is the risk of not having the test?', and 'What are the alternatives?'.

Questions to ask about medications
<http://drkoop.com/wellness/mental_health/medications/page_372_961.asp>

The DrKoop.com site has produced a simple page of questions to which everyone should seek answers before taking any medication.

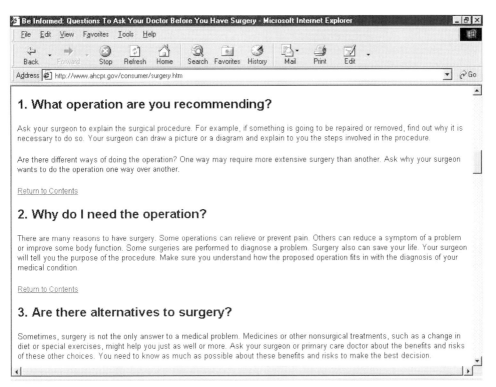

Fig. 12.2   Informing yourself prior to surgery

Presenting information effectively

Writing in a recent issue of the newsletter *He@lth Information on the Internet*, GP Harry Brown spoke of a new syndrome that is spreading fast amongst his patients, known as Internet Printout Syndrome (IPS). Likely candidates can be identified by the 'thick wad of printouts, downloaded from the Internet' they bring to the consultation <http://www.rsm.ac.uk/hii/issue13.pdf>.

Faced with this scenario, Brown suggests that the reaction of most doctors will be a mix of:

- irritation – having to spend time dealing with these printouts;
- hostility – the patient has questioned what the doctor has said;
- rejection – everything on the Internet is rubbish;
- fear – the patient knows more than the doctor.

You do not have to be particularly skilled in people-management and psychology to appreciate that these reactions are not conducive to creating the right environment for an effective dialogue with your doctor. Doctors are only human and anyone who arranges a consultation with the aim of telling the

Table 12.2   Asking the right questions – disease-specific

AIDS – questions to ask your doctor
<http://www.zerit.com/treatment/questions.html>
Though published by a commercial site (Zerit is a drug manufactured by Bristol Myers-Squibb and used in the management of HIV) the questions here are general in nature and do not attempt to steer the patient to any specific form of therapy.

Asthma – questions to ask your doctor
<http://healthatoz.com/atoz/asthma/questions.asp>
In the UK, asthma affects more than 3 million people. Though as yet there is no known cure, there are highly effective ways to control asthma symptoms. The healthAtoZ Web site provides a list of questions asthma patients should seek answers to.

Cancer – questions to ask your doctor
<http://cancernet.nci.nih.gov/wyntk_pubs/cancer.htm#14>
The US National Cancer Institute has produced a general guide to help cancer patients prepare for treatment. For questions that pertain to a particular type of cancer, the following Web sites will be of use:

- Brain tumour <http://www.abta.org/information/questions.htm>
- Breast cancer <http://www.babylonbreastcancer.org/questions.html>
- Lung cancer <http://cancernet.nci.nih.gov/wyntk_pubs/lung.htm#15>
- Ovarian cancer <http://ovarian-news.com/docques_over.html>
- Prostate cancer <http://www.prostate.com/whattoask_pc.htm>
- Testicular cancer <http://www.acor.org/diseases/TC/quest.html>

Diabetes – questions to ask your doctor
<http://ndep.nih.gov/materials/pubs/7-principles/7-english.htm>
The Web site of the National Diabetes Education Programme contains a list of questions diabetic patients should ask their doctor so as to develop a treatment plan that works for them (Fig.12.3).

Heart and stroke – questions to ask your doctor
<http://www.americanheart.org/Heart_and_Stroke_A_Z_Guide/q2ayd.html>
The American Heart Association has produced a comprehensive set of questions that patients who have a heart disease or have suffered a stroke should ask their doctor. To help navigate to the right questions, the page is divided into a number of sections that focus on specific topics such as pacemakers ('How long do the batteries last?', 'Can I still go swimming?') and recovery after a heart attack ('How soon can I drive?' 'How soon can I have sex?').

Mental illness – questions to ask your doctor
<http://sr7.xoom.com/Digdin/questions.html>
The National Alliance for the Mentally Ill has produced a series of questions that people with a mental illness may wish to ask their doctor. Questions cover medication, lifestyle and long-term consequences.

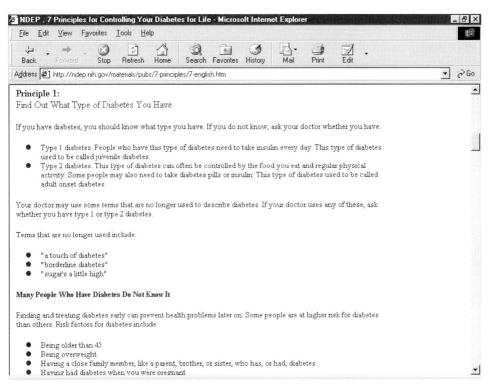

Fig. 12.3 National Diabetes Education Programme – developing a treatment plan

doctor their job – 'I have this condition and need to be treated with this form of therapy' – is unlikely to get very far. Always remember that you are going to see the doctor to ask for *their* professional advice – not to tell them how to treat you.

Having said this, there will be times when you will find information on the Internet that you want to discuss with your doctor. The trick, therefore, is to present this information in a way that the doctor will find least threatening and most useful. Table 12.3 provides a list of "do's" and "don'ts" with regard to presenting your research to your doctor.

Further information and advice on the issue of the doctor/patient relationship can be found at the Doctor Patient Partnership Web site <http://www.doctorpatient.org.uk/> and the Patient's Association Web site <http://www.patients-association.com/intro.htm>.

Conclusion

Though the Internet may have been around in its earliest form since the late 1960s, for most people access from home has become a possibility only within

Table 12.3   Presenting research to the doctor – some "do's" and "don'ts"

DO

✓ Prepare a list of written questions based on your research – make a copy for your doctor.

✓ Prioritise your appointment objectives – a typical consultation lasts less than 10 minutes. Make sure you ask the most important questions first.

✓ If you suspect (or know) that your doctor is highly sceptical about the Internet try introducing information you have found with phrases like 'this information is from a non-profit /government-sponsored organisation …'

✓ Send copies of the **most important** Web pages/articles that you want to discuss with your doctor in *advance* of the consultation, with a brief explanatory note. Highlight the most relevant sections so your doctor can quickly assess this information.

✓ Critically appraise the information you find before mailing it to your doctor.

✓ Know your sources. When discussing something you have found on the Internet your doctor will almost certainly ask for details of authorship. If you can identify the author and the source, the information will be more credible.

✓ Be assertive and polite.

DON'T

✕ Assume everything you find on the Internet is true.

✕ Go to the consultation armed with printouts. These will simply act as a distraction that will impact on the time you have to seek answers to your high priority questions.

✕ Send your doctor everything you can find on the Internet about your condition. They will not have time to read it and may feel that you are trying to tell them their job.

✕ Tell the doctor their job.

✕ Appear too knowledgeable. If you appear to know everything the doctor is telling you they may assume that you know all the pertinent facts and thus to save time may fail to disclose something of which you are not aware.

✕ Be aggressive.

the last four or five years. As this technology is still relatively new, access is still not universal. And, though connectivity amongst doctors is much higher than in the population at large – estimates suggest that 84% of doctors have access to the Internet, compared with a national average of 33% – there are still a significant number of doctors who do not use the Internet. Patients need to be alert to this and sensitive to the fact that they may have access to a greater range of information than that available to the doctor.

It should also be borne in mind that the patient might only have one condition to investigate and can spend as much time as they can afford on researching this topic. Indeed, it is generally recognised that people who participate in self-help groups, for example, become recognised experts in their specific subject. In contrast, a doctor – especially a general practitioner – is required to know enough information about the many hundreds of diseases that can affect us, so as to make an informed decision. There is no way anyone can be an expert on everything.

In this new information age the boundaries between the doctor and the patient are shifting. A recent article in the *Medical Journal of Australia* welcomed the fact that the Internet provides the opportunity for the patient to take more responsibility for their own health care and urges all doctors to 'embrace the concept of the informed patient and to use their web surfing skills' <http://www.mja.com.au/public/issues/xmas98/pemberton/pemberton.html>.

The overall balance in the doctor/patient relationship, however, is maintained by the fact that the doctor is the one who is qualified in assessing the quality and, more importantly, the *relevance* of any information. Using the resources and tips discussed in this chapter the patient and their doctor can enjoy a fruitful relationship based on mutual trust and respect.

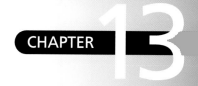

The future

Introduction

A recent report in the *Guardian* newspaper (16 November 2000) painted a picture of the future where we would all be wearing wireless Internet-aware devices that monitored our health and alerted us if something were amiss.

Though this may sound like the stuff of science fiction, there are already products on the market that offer this type of service. Asthma sufferers, for example, can already purchase equipment to monitor their breathing. What makes this equipment unique is the fact that the recorded data can be uploaded (via the Internet) to the manufacturer's Web site where it is then converted into a series of graphs and tables that can help users spot the 'triggers' that might be causing their disease. With the user's permission this data can also be forwarded to the appropriate healthcare team. [Details of this service are available at: <http://www.lifechart.com/webpage_templates/tertiary.php3?page_name=asth_monitor>.]

In addition to disease-specific applications it is increasingly likely that the Internet will offer a means of delivering remote consultations. As broadband Internet connectivity becomes the norm, the facility to hold a remote interactive teleconference with any doctor will become more feasible.

The Internet will also play a growing role in training tomorrow's doctors and in providing them with better administrative services (electronic patient records, online hospital appointment systems etc) and access to computerised decision support systems.

This chapter provides a brief overview of these developments and considers what future role the Internet will play in the delivery of health care.

Telemedicine

Telemedicine can be defined as the use of telecommunication technologies to facilitate the delivery of health care. Though its origins can be traced back to the 1920s – when ship-to-shore radios were used by doctors to assist with medical emergencies at sea – telemedicine has now evolved to the extent that remote doctor/patient and doctor/doctor encounters can take place over the Internet.

In it simplest form the Internet may be used to send information – X-rays, ECG tracings etc – by e-mail, from one doctor to another. This can be particularly useful where local expertise is unavailable or when a second opinion is sought. For example, health professionals who wish to call on the expertise of the US Armed Forces Institute of Pathology (AFIP) <http://www.afip.org/telepathology> can send pathological images by e-mail, or upload them directly on to a secure Web server. Once the image has been received AFIP aims to report the final diagnosis to the referring pathologist within 24 hours.

A considerably more advanced use of telemedicine is remote robotic surgery. A recent study, published in the medical journal the *Annals of Academic Medicine Singapore,* described the case of a patient in Singapore who was operated on by a laparoscopic surgeon located in the US <http://www.ncbi.nlm.nih.gov/entrez/query.fcgi?cmd=Retrieve&db=PubMed &list_uids=11126706&dopt=Abstract>.

One of the more innovative UK telemedicine projects is the eMum service being developed by the Oxford Maternal Infant Care Research and Telemonitoring Centre <http://www.medicine.ox.ac.uk/ndog/tmr/eMum.htm>. This service enables health professionals to monitor remotely the health status of pregnant women (and their unborn children). Information about the mother's health – such as heart rate and blood pressure – is recorded and sent, via the Internet, to a member of the appropriate healthcare team.

Details of other UK-based telemedicine projects can be accessed via the Telemedicine Information Service, a database developed by the University of Portsmouth and the British Library <http://www.tis.bl.uk/>.

Looking ahead, it is likely that telemedical applications will continue to be developed and as broadband technologies become more widespread the virtual consultation will become a feasible alternative. Though UK citizens could benefit from such systems, the greatest impact will be felt in those countries where the population is more widely dispersed or where the health-care system may not be so well developed. Indeed, Internet-based telemedicine is already being used to counter the chronic shortage of doctors in sub-Saharan Africa. Using a system known as SatelLife <http://www.healthnet.org/> local doctors use the Internet to e-mail electrocardiograms, X-ray films etc for analysis and diagnosis to better-equipped and more experienced doctors in the developed world.

Continuing medical education

The various scandals that have rocked the NHS over the past two years – Bristol, Alder-Hey etc – have seriously undermined confidence in the health service. Not surprisingly therefore, there has been a growing call for the introduction of a system that would require all doctors to demonstrate actively that they are fit to practise. In response to this the General Medical Council – the body responsible for licensing doctors in the UK – has announced plans to introduce a mandatory revalidation scheme for doctors <http://www.gmc-uk.org/revalidation/bgrndfrm.htm>.

One of the key components to revalidation will be a requirement for doctors to maintain a portfolio of information about their performance, part of which must identify 'the steps the doctor is taking to stay up to date and to develop professionally'. Using the Internet as a medium for receiving continuing medical education (CME) is one way doctors will realise this objective.

The Internet offers the potential for all health professionals to have access to online courses and training materials. More significantly, these can be accessed at a time and place that is convenient to the user.

Already numerous medical conferences are broadcast over the Internet, thereby allowing the professional to enjoy the benefits of an international conference, without incurring the costs (both financially and in time) of attendance at a real meeting. Indeed, recognising the benefits of the virtual meeting, a number of conferences *only* exist in the virtual environment. Details of these can be found at the Virtual Medical Conference Centre <http://www.vmcc.com/about.html>. Figure 13.1 shows part of an online conference on congestive heart failure, hosted by Dukes University in the US.

Learning on the Internet is not restricted to online courses. The Manchester Visualisation Centre, for example, has produced a number of interactive tools that can be used to practise surgical techniques and operations, including lumbar puncture <http://synaptic.mvc.mcc.ac.uk/Lumbar.html> and ventricular catheterisation <http://synaptic.mvc.mcc.ac.uk/Ventricular_audio.html>.

Other interactive teaching resources include the Trauma Moulage <http://www.trauma.org/resus/moulage/moulage.html>, and the Virtual Autopsy <http://www.le.ac.uk/pathology/teach/va2/index.html>. At the former site you are presented with various scenarios where you have a patient to assess and manage appropriately. In contrast, the Virtual Autopsy site teaches medical students how to identify the cause of death, using images of patient organs and post-mortem reports.

Online, interactive services such as those described here not only make the process of learning more enjoyable, but also more effective. One study that compared a Web-based self-study module with a printed self-study module concluded that online tutorials 'produce greater learning efficiency and

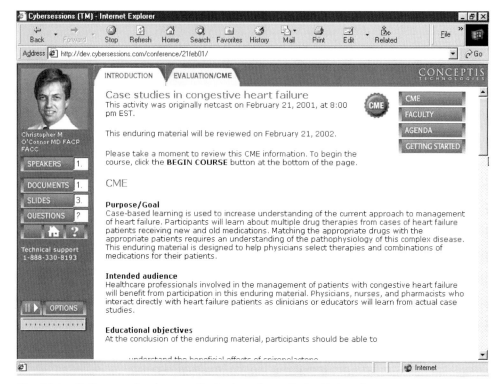

Fig. 13.1 Online continuing medical education – Duke University

satisfaction than print materials' <http://www.ncbi.nlm.nih.gov/entrez/query.fcgi?cmd=Retrieve&db=PubMed&list_uids=10858176&dopt=Abstract>.

The Internet provides opportunities for all health professionals to further their medical education and keep up to date. In the longer term this will lead to a better-trained and more able workforce that, in turn, can deliver patient care more effectively.

The interactive health service

The Internet also allows for the core administrative health services to be delivered more effectively. In the UK the *NHS Plan: a plan for investment, a plan for reform* <http://www.nhs.uk/nhsplan> highlights the commitment of the UK government to invest in information technology to deliver 'services faster and more conveniently for patients'. Specific objectives include:

- enabling doctors to access electronic personal medical records by 2004;
- the introduction of electronic prescribing of medicines by 2004;
- the development of an electronic appointment booking system by 2005.

Consequently, in the near future when you visit your GP (or indeed, any GP anywhere in the country) he/she will be able to access your medical records online. In the event that a hospital appointment (or specialist referral) is deemed necessary your GP will be able to arrange this online, whilst you are still at the surgery, thereby ensuring that the appointment allocated is at a convenient time. If a prescription is required the GP will be able to e-mail this request to a local pharmacy where, if the drug is immediately available, it will be ready for you to collect on your way home.

In the longer term these services will be extended and patients will be able to access their personal medical records – via smart cards – and communicate directly (by e-mail and video-conferencing) with healthcare professionals.

In parallel with these developments it seems increasingly likely that health professionals will turn to the Internet to access computerised decision-support systems (DSS). DSS are used to help minimise the incidence of misdiagnosis and ensure that best practices are adhered to.

The American Thoracic Society in association with the US Centers for Disease Control have developed an Internet-based DSS to help doctors apply the correct preventive therapy for patients infected with tuberculosis (TB). Though

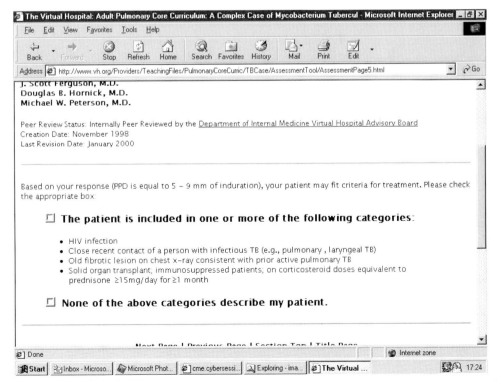

Fig. 13.2   Online decision support systems

these guidelines are accessible in paper form, they are complex to use and as a consequence many clinicians find them 'challenging to apply'. The Web-based system <http:/www.vh.org/Providers/TeachingFiles/PulmonaryCoreCurric/TBCase/AssessmentTool/AssessmentPage1.html> delivers patient-specific recommendations based on real data supplied by the clinician (Fig. 13.2).

One scenario-based study that looked at the effectiveness of this computerised system found that the correct treatment – as validated by independent experts – was given in 95% of cases. When the same scenarios were put to doctors who only had access to the paper guidelines, fewer than 57% recommended treatment that adhered to the best practice guidelines. This certainly suggests that DSS have considerable value in the healthcare environment.

Other Internet-based DSS include one for asthma management <http:/www.vh.org/Providers/ClinGuide/AsthmaIM/Default.html> as well as the more general computerised medical diagnosis service, DXplain <http://www.lcs.mgh.harvard.edu/>. In this latter case a range of clinical findings – signs, symptoms and data from laboratory tests – is used to produce a ranked list of diagnoses.

Using the Internet as the distribution method for DSS ensures that all doctors have equal access to these tools, and by virtue of the fact that no special software is required (they all work through a standard Web browser) professionals can start to use these services with minimal training.

Endpiece

The size and volatility of the Internet means that any book on this topic can never be anything more than a snapshot of what is available. New resources appear and, more frustratingly, established ones change or simply disappear in the void of cyberspace.

To help minimise the frustration this causes, many of the Web sites discussed and referenced in this book can be accessed from *The Patient's Internet Handbook* Web site <http://www.patient-handbook.co.uk>. If we become aware that a site has moved we will endeavour to find its new location and publish its new address on the Web site.

You can also use this site to contact the authors with any questions you have about the book, or to suggest items or topics for inclusion in any future edition.

We look forward to hearing from you.

100 medical conditions: sources of information on the Internet

Overview

We hope that having read the preceding chapters you will now be equipped to find and evaluate health information on the Internet. However, as a starting point, we have selected 100 medical conditions and, for each one, provided a map to the key Internet information sources. For each condition we have identified a support group and provided full contact details. We have also identified relevant discussion lists and newsgroups and suggested summary documents that provide an overview of the condition or disease.

Support groups

Support groups are a great source of information, expertise and help. In this directory we have, where possible, identified the most specific group. For example, in the case of breast cancer, we were able to select the group Breast Cancer Care. For bladder cancer, however, we could not identify a specific group so an alternative is suggested. As this is a guide to Web resources, we also tended only to include those groups that have an active Web site.

Discussion lists and newsgroups

As highlighted in Chapter 6, discussion lists and newsgroups provide the opportunity for health consumers to communicate with fellow patients throughout the world and in so doing seek first-hand help, advice and support.

In addition to providing the name of the discussion forum and joining details we have also tried to identify whether an archive of messages is available on the Web. These can be particularly useful in helping to determine whether or not a specific forum meets your needs.

Suggested summary documents

Finally, for each condition we have identified two or three useful Web documents, from trustworthy sources, which give a brief overview or an introduction to the condition. In selecting these documents we looked first to UK-based sites and then supplemented them with other material, mainly American.

Acne

Support group

Acne Support Group
PO Box 230
Hayes
Middlesex
UB4 0UT

Tel: 020 8561 6868
Fax: 020 8845 5424
E-mail: n/a
Web page: <http://www.m2w3.com/acne/> and <http://www.stopspots.org/>

Online discussion list

Name of list: **eczemapsoriasis**

The list has been set up to offer support to anyone suffering from skin disorders, and for everyone who is interested to learn about the causes, prevention and treatment for acne, dermatitis, and other skin disorders.

To join this discussion list send a blank message:

To: eczemapsoriasis-subscribe@yahoogroups.com
Text: leave blank

Web archive of messages: for members only. More information available at: <http://groups.yahoo.com/group/ECZEMAPSORIASIS>.

Online newsgroup

Name of newsgroup: <news://alt.skincare.acne>

To view the Web archive of messages, go to <http://groups.google.com/> and enter the following: alt.skincare.acne

Suggested summary documents

An acne information sheet, authored by the Royal College of General Practitioners, providing an overview of this condition is available at: <http://www.rcgp.org.uk/faculty/severn/s18.htm>.

For a more in-depth and up-to-date document see the 'Questions and answers about acne', published by the US National Institute of Arthritis and Musculoskeletal and Skin Diseases at: <http://www.nih.gov/niams/healthinfo/acne/acne.htm>.

Acquired Immune Deficiency Syndrome (AIDS)

See also **Sexually transmitted diseases.**

Support group
Terrence Higgins Trust
52–54 Grays Inn Road
London
WC1X 8JU

Tel (Helpline): 020 7242 1010
Tel: 020 7831 0330
Fax: 020 7242 0121
E-mail: info@tht.org.uk
Web page: <http://www.tht.org.uk>

Online discussion lists
Yahoo! Groups hosts over 270 discussion lists relating to AIDS and HIV. To see a list of them, point your Web browser at: <http://dir.groups.yahoo.com/dir/1600061590>.

One forum that deals with all aspects of protease-inhibitor treatment, including side effects, lifestyle changes, and drug interactions, is the **PI-TREAT** list. To subscribe to this list visit the following site and complete the online joining form: <http://www.pozlink.com/>.

Online newsgroup
Name of newsgroup: <news://misc.health.aids>

To view the Web archive of messages, go to <http://groups.google.com/> and enter the following: misc.health.aids

Suggested summary documents
The US National Institute of Allergy and Infectious Diseases has produced a detailed fact sheet about HIV and AIDS. This is available at: <http://www.niaid.nih.gov/factsheets/hivinf.htm>.

For a UK perspective, the AIDS Education and Research Trust (AVERT) has produced a detailed list of frequently asked questions, with answers. This can be read at: <http://www.avert.org/faq1.htm>.

Alcoholism

Support group
Alcoholics Anonymous
General Service Office of AA
PO Box 1
Stonebow House
Stonebow
York
Y01 2NJ

Tel (Helpline): 020 7833 0022
Tel: 01904 644026
Fax: 01904 629091
E-mail: n/a
Web page: <http://www.alcoholics-anonymous.org.uk/>

Online discussion lists
A great number of lists exist for people with alcohol problems, many of which are highly specific. For example, the list ADDL looks specifically at the consequences of drinking and driving. One of the more general lists is **alcohol-l**.

To join this discussion list send the following message:

To: listproc@lists.missouri.edu
Text: subscribe alcohol-l *firstname lastname*

Web archive of messages: not available.

Online newsgroup
Name of newsgroup: <news://alt.recovery.addiction.alcoholism>

To view the Web archive of messages, go to <http://groups.google.com/> and enter the following: alt.recovery.addiction.alcoholism

Suggested summary documents
The US National Institute on Alcohol Abuse and Alcoholism has produced a 12-page guide entitled 'The physicians' guide to helping patients with alcohol problems', available at:
<http://silk.nih.gov/silk/niaaa1/publication/physicn.htm>.

In the UK, the Institute of Alcohol Studies has produced a number of useful fact sheets, all of which can be downloaded from:
<http://www.ias.org.uk/factsheets/default.htm>.

Alzheimer's disease

Support group

Alzheimer's Disease Society
Gordon House
10 Greencoat Place
London
SW1P 9PH

Tel (Helpline): 0845 300 0336
Tel: 020 7306 0606
Fax: 020 7306 0808
E-mail: info@alzheimers.org.uk
Web page: <http://www.alzheimers.org.uk/>

Online discussion list

Name of list: **alzheimer**

The **alzheimer** list is an educational service created and sponsored by the Washington University Alzheimer's Disease Research Center (ADRC) in St Louis, Missouri supported, in part, by a grant from the National Institute on Aging (NIA).

To join this discussion list send the following message:

To: majordomo@wubios.wustl.edu
Text: subscribe alzheimer *firstname lastname*

Web archive of messages available at:
<http://www.adrc.wustl.edu/ALZHEIMER/>

Online newsgroup

Name of newsgroup: <news://alt.support.alzheimers>

To view the Web archive of messages, go to <http://groups.google.com/> and enter the following: alt.support.alzheimers

Suggested summary documents

The UK Alzheimer's Disease Society has a number of useful documents on its Web site <http://www.alzheimers.org/uk>, as does the UK-based Web site emental-health.com. Information about Alzheimer's can be found at: <http://www.emental-health.com/alzheimer.htm>.

The US National Institute of Neurological Disorders and Stroke has an excellent 'mini-information sheet' that provides clear answers to the most frequently-asked questions such as 'What is Alzheimer's disease?', 'Is there any treatment?' and 'What is the prognosis?'. This document is available at: <http://www.ninds.nih.gov/health_and_medical/disorders/alzheimers disease_doc.htm>.

For a more detailed overview, the resources at the Alzheimer's Disease Education and Referral (ADEAR) Center's Web site <http://www.alzheimers.org/> can be consulted.

Angina

Support group
British Heart Foundation
14 Fitzhardinge Street
London
W1H 4DH

Heart Health Line: 0870 600 6566
Tel: 020 7935 0185
Fax: 020 7486 5820
E-mail: n/a
Web page: <http://www.bhf.org.uk/>

Online discussion list
Name of list: **hearttalk-l**

A discussion list and support group for patients with heart disease.

To join this discussion list send the following message:

To: listserv@maelstrom.stjohns.edu
Text: subscribe hearttalk-l *firstname lastname*

Web archive of messages available at:
<http://maelstrom.stjohns.edu/archives/hearttalk-l.html>

Online newsgroup
Name of newsgroup: <news://alt.support.heart-defects>

To view the Web archive of messages, go to <http://groups.google.com/> and enter the following: alt.support.heart-defects

Suggested summary documents

The US National Heart, Lung and Blood Institute has produced a brief 'Facts about angina' document, available at: <http://www.nhlbi.nih.gov/health/public/heart/other/angina.htm>. Further information can be found at the site of the American Academy of Family Physicians <http://www.aafp.org/patientinfo/angina.html>.

Though not aimed specifically at patients the Health Evidence Bulletin (Wales) Web site has a very useful summary relating to the effective care and management of stable and unstable angina. This can be accessed at: <http://hebw.uwcm.ac.uk/cardio/index.html>.

Ankylosing spondylitis

Support group
National Ankylosing Spondylitis Society
PO Box 179
Mayfield
East Sussex
TN20 6ZL

Tel: 01435 873527
Fax: 01435 873027
E-mail: nass@nass.co.uk
Web page: <http://nass.co.uk>

Online discussion list
Name of list: **risg-l**

An information and support group for people who themselves have or are close to people who have arthritic afflictions such as Reiter's syndrome and/or ankylosing spondylitis.

To join this discussion list send the following message:

To: listserv@home.ease.lsoft.com
Text: subscribe risg-l *firstname lastname*

Web archive of messages available at:
<http://home.ease.lsoft.com/archives/risg-l.html>

Online newsgroup
Name of newsgroup: <news://alt.support.arthritis>

To view the Web archive of messages, go to <http://groups.google.com/> and enter the following: alt.support.arthritis

Suggested summary document

The Spondylitis Association of America has produced a number of quick guides to this condition, including 'What is spondylitis?', 'What are the symptoms, diagnosis and treatment?' and 'What complications can arise?'. All these guides can be downloaded from: <http://www.spondylitis.org/faq.htm>.

The Arthritis Research Campaign has also produced a useful booklet on this condition. This can be accessed at: <http://www.arc.org.uk/about_arth/booklets/31_as_92-1.htm>.

Anorexia nervosa

Support group

Eating Disorders Association
1st Floor, Wensum House
103 Prince of Wales Road
Norwich
Norfolk
NR1 1DW

Tel (Helpline): 01603 621414
Tel (Admin): 01603 619090
Fax: 01603 664915
E-mail: info@edauk.com
Web page: <http://www.edauk.com/>

Online discussion list

Name of list: **ased-list**

A supportive mailing list for people with eating disorders – including anorexia, bulimia, binge eating, compulsive overeating, and emotional eating problems.

To join this discussion list send the following message:

To: majordomo@samurai.com
Text: subscribe ased-list

Web archive of messages: not available.

Online newsgroup

Name of newsgroup: <news://alt.support.eating-disord>

To view the Web archive of messages, go to <http://groups.google.com/> and enter the following: alt.support.eating-disord

Suggested summary documents

The Royal College of Psychiatrists has produced a clearly written and authoritative anorexia fact-sheet. This can be accessed at: <http://www.rcpsych.ac.uk/public/help/anor/anor_frame.htm>.

For information about the emotional impact on the sufferer and their friends and family see 'Talking about eating disorders' produced by the Health Education Board for Scotland. This is available at: <http://www.hebs.scot.nhs.uk/mental/mntpeat.htm>.

Anxiety

Support group

First Steps to Freedom
7 Avon Court
School Lane
Kenilworth
Warwickshire
CV8 2GX

Tel: 01926 864473
Fax: 0870 164 0567
E-mail: info@firststeps.demon.co.uk
Web page: <http://www.firststeps.demon.co.uk/>

Online discussion list

There are at least 32 online discussion lists that deal with anxiety (see: <http://www.topica.com/dir/?cid=2295>). One of the more general lists is the **anx-dis** list.

Name of list: **anx-dis**

To join this discussion list send the following message:

To: anx-dis@maelstrom.stjohns.edu
Text: subscribe anx-dis

Web archive of messages available at:
<http://maelstrom.stjohns.edu/archives/anx-dis.html>

Online newsgroup

Name of newsgroup: <news://alt.support.anxiety-panic>

To view the Web archive of messages, go to <http://groups.google.com/> and enter the following: alt.support.anxiety-panic

Suggested summary documents

The US National Institute of Mental Health provides a wealth of resources that focus on specific anxiety disorders including post traumatic stress, obsessive compulsive and phobias. To access this information, go to: <http://www.nimh.nih.gov/anxiety/anxiety/index.htm>.

The UK Support group the Mental Health Foundation has also produced a quick guide to anxiety, that considers the causes of stress and how it can be managed. This document is available at: <http://www.mentalhealth.org.uk/factanx.htm>.

Arthritis

Support group

Arthritis Care
18 Stephenson Way
London
NW1 2HD

Tel (Helpline): 0800 289170
Tel: 020 7916 1500
Fax: 020 7916 1505
E-mail: n/a
Web page: <http://www.arthritiscare.org.uk/>

Online discussion list

Name of list: **arthritis**

A general discussion list for arthritis sufferers.

To join this discussion list send the following message:

To: arthritis@maelstrom.stjohns.edu
Text: subscribe arthritis

Web archive of messages available at:
<http://maelstrom.stjohns.edu/archives/arthritis.html>

Online newsgroup

Name of newsgroup: <news://alt.support.arthritis>

To view the Web archive of messages, go to <http://groups.google.com/> and enter the following: alt.support.arthritis

Suggested summary documents

The Arthritis Research Campaign (ARC) Web site offers a great deal of information about arthritis – including 60 online booklets that deal both with very general topics such as 'What is arthritis', through to highly specialised guides including 'Gardening with arthritis' and 'Arthritis: sexual aspects and parenthood'. The ARC also provides information about the prevalence of arthritis and details of current and ongoing research. All this information can be reached from: <http://www.arc.org.uk/about_arth/chome.htm>.

Asthma

Support group

National Asthma Campaign
Providence House
Providence Place
London
N1 0NT

Tel (Helpline): 0845 7010203
Tel: 020 7226 2260
Fax: 020 7704 0740
E-mail: n/a
Web page: <http://www.asthma.org.uk/>

Online discussion list

Name of list: **asthma-l**

A general discussion list for asthma sufferers.

To join this discussion list send the following message:

To: asthma-l@maelstrom.stjohns.edu
Text: subscribe asthma-l

Web archive of messages available at:
<http://maelstrom.stjohns.edu/archives/asthma-l.html>

Online newsgroup

Name of newsgroup: <news://alt.support.asthma>

To view the Web archive of messages, go to <http://groups.google.com/> and enter the following: alt.support.asthma

Suggested summary documents

The National Asthma Campaign has produced a quick summary guide to asthma in a question and answer format. This is available at: <http://www.asthma.org.uk/what.html>.

For more detailed information the US National Heart, Blood and Lung Institute has authored a number of booklets including 'Controlling your asthma' and 'Asthma and physical activity in school'. These can be found at: <http://www.nhlbi.nih.gov/health/public/lung/index.htm>.

Attention deficit disorder with hyperactivity (ADDH/ADHD)

Support group

ADD/ADHD Family Support Group
1a The High Street
Dilton Marsh
Nr. Westbury
Wiltshire
BA13 4DL

Tel (Helpline): 01380 726710
Tel: 01373 826045
Fax: 01373 825158
E-mail: n/a
Web page: <http://www.pncl.co.uk/~prospero/adhd.html>

Online discussion list

Name of list: **addparents**

A discussion list for support and information sharing for parents who have children with attention deficit/hyperactivity disorder (ADHD).

To join this discussion list send the following message:

To: listserver@ourfriends.com
Text: subscribe addparents

Web archive of messages: not available.

Online newsgroup
Name of newsgroup: <news://alt.support.attn-deficit>

To view the Web archive of messages, go to <http://groups.google.com/> and enter the following: alt.support.attn-deficit

Suggested summary documents
The US National Institute of Mental Health has produced an online booklet on ADDH that considers the symptoms as well as current treatment options. This is available at: <http://www.nimh.nih.gov/publicat/adhd.cfm>.

Another excellent overview is provided in an online article in the magazine *Scientific American*. Published in 1998 this article looks at causes and treatment options and provides links to a number of related pieces. This article can be found at:
<http://www.sciam.com/1998/0998issue/0998barkley.html>.

Autism

Support group
National Autistic Society
393 City Road
London
EC1V 1NG

Tel: 020 7833 2299
Fax: 020 7833 9666
E-mail: nas@nas.org.uk
Web page: <http://www.oneworld.org/autism_uk/>

Online discussion list
Name of list: **Autism and Developmental Disabilities**

To join this discussion list send the following message:

To: autism@maelstrom.stjohns.edu
Text: subscribe autism *firstname lastname*

Web archive of messages available at: <http://web.syr.edu/~rjkopp/autdigest.html>

Online newsgroup
Name of newsgroup: <news://alt.support.autism>

To view the Web archive of messages, go to <http://groups.google.com/> and enter the following: alt.support.autism

Suggested summary documents

The National Autistic Society's Web site contains a wealth of information about this condition. Included here is a range of fact sheets, plus detailed information on current therapies and interventions, and articles on the educational needs of children with autism. This information is available at: <http://www.oneworld.org/autism_uk/factsheet/factsh.html>.

Back pain

Support group

Back Care
16 Elmtree Road
Teddington
Middlesex
TW11 8ST

Tel: 020 8977 5474
Fax: 020 8943 5318
E-mail: back_pain@compuserve.com
Web page: <http://www.backpain.org/>

Online discussion list

Name of list: **pain-l**

Though not limited *exclusively* to the problem of back pain, this list has much comment and discussion on the subject. To join this discussion list send the following message:

To: listserv@maelstrom.stjohns.edu
Text: subscribe pain-l *firstname lastname*

Web archive of messages available at:
<http://maelstrom.stjohns.edu/archives/pain-l.html>

A more focused list is the **Support – Back Pain** list. To join this discussion list send the following message:

To: vtg1221-subscribe@topica.com
Text: leave blank

Online newsgroup

Name of newsgroup: <news://alt.support.chronic.pain>

To view the Web archive of messages, go to <http://groups.google.com/> and enter the following: alt.support.chronic.pain

Suggested summary documents

The Arthritis Research Campaign has produced a useful online booklet on backache, that covers issues such as symptoms, diagnosis and treatment as well as posing (and answering) a number of frequently asked questions. This booklet can be read at:
<http://www.arc.org.uk/about_arth/booklets/35_back_93-1.htm>.

In the US, the Agency for Healthcare Research and Quality has produced a more detailed guide entitled 'Understanding acute low back problems'. This document looks at both conservative and surgical methods of treating low back pain. This document is available at:
<http://text.nlm.nih.gov/ftrs/pick?collect=ahcpr&dbName=lbpp&cd=1&t=958497252>.

Bedwetting

See **Enuresis**

Bereavement

Support group

Cruse Bereavement Care UK
Cruse House
126 Sheen Road
Richmond
Surrey
TW9 1UR

Tel (Bereavement Line): 020 8332 7227
Tel: 020 8940 4818
Fax: 020 8940 7638
E-mail: n/a
Web page: Only local branches seem to have Web sites. eg: Darlington at:
<http://www.aeiou.co.uk/cruse/>

Online discussion list

There are many discussion lists related to death, grief and bereavement. Many of these are very specific, such as **grief-parents-neonate**, set up for parents who have had a child die from miscarriage, stillbirth, or neonatal death. A fairly comprehensive list of these groups can be accessed at: <http://www.topica.com/dir/?cid=242>.

A more general discussion list is simply called **grief**

Name of list: **grief**

To join this discussion list send the following message:

To: majordomo@listserv.prodigy.com
Text: subscribe grief *your e-mail address*

Web archive of messages: Not available.

Online newsgroup

Name of newsgroup: <news://alt.support.grief>

To view the Web archive of messages, go to <http://groups.google.com/> and enter the following: alt.support.grief

Suggested summary documents

The Royal College of Psychiatrists has written a brief fact sheet on bereavement that discusses common feelings such as anger and guilt. This can be downloaded from: <http://www.rcpsych.ac.uk/public/help/bereav/bereavem.htm>.

In the US the Nemours Foundation has produced a number of online leaflets including 'How to help your child deal with death' <http://kidshealth.org/parent/emotions/feelings/death.html> and 'When somebody dies' <http://kidshealth.org/kid/feeling/somedie.html>.

Bipolar disorder (manic depression)

Support groups

Manic Depression Fellowship
Castle Works
21 St George's Road
London
SE1 6ES

Tel: 020 7793 2600
Fax: 020 7793 2639
E-mail: mdf@mdf.org.uk
Web page: <http://www.mdf.org.uk/>

Two other useful groups are:
Depression Alliance: <http://www.depressionalliance.org/>
Mind: <http://www.mind.org.uk/>

Online discussion list

Yahoo! Groups hosts over 150 e-mail lists on bipolar disorder. To see a list of them, go to: <http://dir.groups.yahoo.com/dir/1600061749>. One of the largest is:

Name of list: **Bipolar World**

This list has been established for the discussion of bipolar disorder (manic depression) 'in a warm, safe and supportive atmosphere'.

To join this discussion list send the following message:

To: bipolar_world-subscribe@yahoogroups.com
Text: leave blank

Web archive of messages: for members only.

Further information available at:
<http://groups.yahoo.com/group/Bipolar_World>

Online newsgroups

Name of newsgroup: <news://alt.support.depression.manic>
Name of newsgroup: <news://soc.support.depression.manic>

To view the Web archives of messages, go to <http://groups.google.com/> and enter either: alt.support.depression.manic *or* soc.support.depression.manic

Suggested summary documents

The UK-based Web site emental-health.com has a range of information sources on bipolar disorders, available at: <http://www.emental-health.com/bipolar.htm>.

The mental health charity Mind has produced a booklet called 'Understanding manic depression'. To access this point your browser at: <http://www.mind.org.uk/information/information_understanding.asp>.

The US National Institute of Mental Health has produced a clear and detailed guide to bipolar disorder, covering symptoms, causes and treatment. It can be found at: <http://www.nimh.nih.gov/publicat/bipolar.cfm>.

Bladder cancer

See also **Cancer.**

Support group
There is no UK support group specifically for bladder cancer, but there are several cancer support groups, for example:

CancerBACUP
3 Bath Place
Rivington Street
London
EC2A 3JR

Tel (Helpline): 0808 800 1234
Tel: 020 7696 9003
Fax: 020 7696 9002
E-mail: info@cancerbacup.org.uk
Web page: <http://www.cancerbacup.org.uk/>

Online discussion list
Name of list: **bladder-onc**

Part of a large family of oncology lists, this list provides support relating to bladder cancer.

To join this discussion list send the following message:

To: bladder-onc@listserv.acor.org
Text: join bladder-onc

Web archive of messages available at: <http://listserv.acor.org/archives/bladder-onc.html>

Online newsgroup
Name of newsgroup: <news://alt.support.cancer>

To view the Web archive of messages, go to <http://groups.google.com/> and enter the following: alt.support.cancer

Suggested summary documents

The US National Cancer Institute has produced a clear and informative document called 'What You Need to Know About Bladder Cancer' which discusses the typical symptoms, diagnosis and treatment options. This guide can be read at: <http://cancernet.nci.nih.gov/wyntk_pubs/bladder.htm#2>.

As with most cancers, the earlier it is diagnosed the greater the chance that it can be successfully treated. The Mayo Clinic has written a brief guide, 'Early Detection is Crucial', which highlights some of the warning signs everyone should look out for. This article can be found at: <http://www.mayohealth.org/mayo/9803/htm/bladder.htm>.

Blood pressure, high

See **Hypertension.**

Bowel cancer

See **Colorectal cancer.**

Brain cancer

See also **Cancer.**

Support group

UK Brain Tumour Society
22 Cambridge Road
Aldershot
Hampshire
GU11 3JZ

Tel/Fax: 01252 653807
E-mail: give.hope@virgin.net
Web page: <http://freespace.virgin.net/give.hope/guest/ukbts.html>

Online discussion list

Name of list: **head-neck-onc**

Part of a large family of oncology (cancer) lists, this list provides support relating to cancers of the head and neck.

To join this discussion list send the following message:

To: head-neck-onc@listserv.acor.org
Text: subscribe head-neck-onc

Web archive of messages available at: <http://listserv.acor.org/archives/head-neck-onc.html>

Online newsgroup
Name of newsgroup: <news://alt.support.cancer>

To view the Web archive of messages, go to <http://groups.google.com/> and enter the following: alt.support.cancer

Suggested summary documents
As part of its 'What you need to know about' series, the US National Cancer Institute has compiled a useful overview of brain tumours, including causes, symptoms, and treatment options. This guide can be found at: <http://cancernet.nci.nih.gov/wyntk_pubs/brain.htm>.

In the UK the CancerBACUP self-help group has commissioned a number of booklets on brain cancers. Available documents include 'Understanding cancer of the brain' <http://www.cancerbacup.org.uk/info/brain.htm> as well as a number of fact sheets on more specific types of cancer. These include 'Understanding acoustic neuroma' <http://www.cancerbacup.org.uk/info/acousticneuroma.htm> and 'Mixed gliomas' <http://www.cancerbacup.org.uk/info/mixedglioma.htm>. All documents state when the guide was written and last updated.

Breast cancer

See also **Cancer.**

Support groups
Breast Cancer Care
Kiln House
210 New Kings Road
London
SW6 4NZ

Tel: 020 7384 2984
Fax: 020 7384 3387
E-mail: bcc@breastcancercare.org.uk
Web page: <http://www.breastcancercare.org.uk>

See also:
Action Against Breast Cancer: <http://www.aabc.org.uk/>
Breakthrough Breast Cancer:
<http://www.breakthrough.org.uk/docs/home.asp>
Breast Cancer Campaign: <http://www.bcc-uk.org/>

Online discussion list
Name of list: **BRCA**

Part of a large family of oncology (cancer) lists, this list provides various kinds of support relating to cancer of the breast.

To join this discussion list send the following message:

To: listserv@listserv.acor.org
Text: subscribe brca

Web archive of messages available at:
<http://listserv.acor.org/archives/BRCA.html>

Online newsgroup
Name of newsgroup: <news://alt.support.cancer.breast>

To view the Web archive of messages, go to <http://groups.google.com/> and enter the following: alt.support.cancer.breast

Suggested summary documents
The Royal Marsden Hospital has produced clear and helpful patient information leaflets, which provide information about living with and treating different types of cancer. The content is based on common questions asked by patients. All titles are regularly reviewed and updated, and new booklets are added each year. The booklet for breast cancer is available at: <http://www.royalmarsden.org/patientinfo/booklets/breast_cancer/index.asp>.

As part of its excellent booklet series, the charity Cancer BACUP has produced 'Understanding cancer of the breast'. As well as explaining causes, symptoms, diagnosis and treatment, it discusses the emotional shock of a cancer diagnosis, and provides information about useful organisations and 'recommended reading'. It can be found at: <http://www.cancerbacup.org.uk/info/breast.htm>.

Bronchitis

Support group

British Lung Foundation
78 Hatton Garden
London
EC1N 8LD

Tel: 020 7831 5831
Fax: 020 7831 5832
E-mail: bl@britishlungfoundation.com
Web: <http://www.lunguk.org/>

Online discussion list

Name of list: **chronic-obstructive-pulmonary disease**

To join this discussion list complete the Web form at: <http://copd-support.com/join.html>.

Web archive of messages available at: <http://members.boardhost.com/COPD/>

Online newsgroup

Name of newsgroup: <news://alt.support.pulmonary>

To view the Web archive of messages, go to <http://groups.google.com/> and enter the following: alt.support.pulmonary

Suggested summary documents

The American Lung Association has produced a guide to chronic bronchitis which considers the causes and treatments and gives practical advice on what steps you can take to help manage this condition. This guide can be accessed at: <http://www.lungusa.org/diseases/lungchronic.html>.

For further information, the *Respiratory Diseases Bulletin*, part of the Health Evidence Bulletin Wales series, may be consulted. This guide looks at all types of respiratory diseases (asthma, cystic fibrosis, pneumonia etc) and also includes chapters on acute bronchitis and bronchiolitis and the management of bronchitis and emphysema with and without drug therapy. The guide is available at: <http://hebw.uwcm.ac.uk/respdis/index.html>.

Bulimia

Support group

Eating Disorders Association
103 Prince of Wales Road
Norwich
Norfolk
NR1 1DW

Tel: 01603 621414
Fax: 01603 664915
E-mail: info@edauk.com
Web page: <http://www.edauk.com>

Online discussion list

Name of list: **eat-dis**

To join this discussion list complete the Web form at:
<http://maelstrom.stjohns.edu/archives/eat-dis.html>.

Web archive of messages available at:
<http://maelstrom.stjohns.edu/archives/eat-dis.html>

Online newsgroup

Name of newsgroup: <news://alt.support.eating-disord>

To view the Web archive of messages, go to <http://groups.google.com/> and
enter the following: alt.support.eating-disord

Suggested summary documents

The US Food and Drug Administration has written a good background
document that gives the clinical definition of bulimia and considers some of
the reasons why people develop eating disorders. This document can be
found at: <htpp://www.fda.gov/opacom/catalog/eatdis.html>.

For information about the emotional impact on the sufferer and their friends
and family, see 'Talking about eating disorders' produced by the Health
Education Board for Scotland. This is available at:
<http://www.hebs.scot.nhs.uk/mental/mntpeat.htm>.

Burns

Support group
American Burn Association
ABA Central Office – Chicago
625 N. Michigan Ave, Ste 1530
Chicago
Illinois 60611
USA

Tel: 001 312 642 9260
Fax: 001 312 642 9130
E-mail: info@ameriburn.org
Web page: <http://ameriburn.org/index.html>

Online discussion list
Name of list: **ABA Online Forum**

Though membership is limited to members of the American Burn Association, postings to the list can be read by anyone.

Web archive of messages available at: <http://ameriburn.org/disc2_frm.htm>

Online newsgroup
Name of newsgroup: <news://alt.support.chronic-pain>

To view the Web archive of messages, go to <http://groups.google.com/> and enter the following: alt.support.chronic-pain

Suggested summary documents
The American Medical Association has produced a fact sheet entitled 'Children with burn injuries' <http://www.ama-assn.org/insight/spec_con/patient/pat082.htm> which provides some basic practical advice on how to prevent burns as well as giving some information on what to do if your child has a major burn.

A more detailed document – and one that was written primarily for health professionals – is the New South Wales 'Management guidelines for people with burn injury'. This document can be downloaded from: <http://www.health.nsw.gov.au/public-health/burns/burnsmgt.html>.

Cancer

Support groups

There are several general nationwide cancer charities, as well as a range of organisations concerned with specific types of cancer. (For more information on specific cancers, see separate entries.) Most of the larger groups have a Web presence:

Cancer BACUP: <http://www.cancerbacup.org.uk/>
Cancer Care Society:
<http://www.cancercaresoc.demon.co.uk/home.html>
Cancer Research Campaign: <http://www.crc.org.uk/>
Marie Curie Cancer Care: <http://www.mariecurie.org.uk/>
Women's Nationwide CCC: <http://www.wnccc.org.uk/>

Online discussion lists

The Association of Cancer Online Resources, Inc (ACOR) is an American charitable organisation which aims to 'provide information and support to cancer patients and those who care for them through the creation and maintenance of cancer-related Internet mailing lists and Web-based resources'.

The list archives can be found at: <http://listserv.acor.org/archives/>.

There are over 120 lists, most specialising in specific forms of cancer. The general list is called **Cancer**; it is an unmoderated discussion list for patients, family, friends, caregivers, researchers and health professionals, set up to discuss clinical/psychosocial issues pertaining to all forms of cancer.

To join this discussion list, send the following message:

To: listserv@listserv.acor.org
Text: subscribe cancer

Web archive of messages available at: <http://listserv.acor.org/archives/cancer.html>

Online newsgroups

There are two newsgroups concerned with cancer:

Name of newsgroup: <news://alt.support.cancer>
Name of newsgroup: <news://sci.med.diseases.cancer>

To view the Web archives of messages, go to <http://groups.google.com/> and enter either: alt.support.cancer *or* sci.med.diseases.cancer

Suggested summary documents

Cancer BACUP has produced an excellent series of online booklets on 'Understanding cancer', which cover causes, symptoms, diagnosis and treatment of most common cancers. Other booklets provide detailed information about cancer treatments and drugs, and about emotional and practical aspects of living with cancer. The booklets are available in full text at <http://www.cancerbacup.org.uk/info/>.

As part of its CancerNet service, the US National Cancer Institute provides detailed information on a range of cancers, including symptoms, treatment and follow-up care. The 'What you need to know about cancer' series is available in full text at: <http://cancernet.nci.nih.gov/wyntk_pubs/>.

For specific cancers covered in this directory

See also **Bladder cancer; Brain cancer; Breast cancer; Cervical cancer; Colorectal cancer; Leukaemia; Lung cancer; Lymphoma; Melanoma; Oral cancer; Ovarian cancer; Pancreatic cancer; Prostate cancer; Stomach cancer; Testicular cancer; Thyroid cancer.**

Carpal tunnel syndrome

Support group

Arthritis Research Campaign
Copeman House
St Mary's Court
St Mary's Gate
Chesterfield
Derbyshire
S41 7TD

Tel: 01246 558033
Fax: 01246 558007
E-mail: info@arc.org.uk
Web page: <http://www.arc.org.uk/common/home.htm>

Online discussion list

Name of list: **Sorehand**

A list set up to discuss issues pertaining to carpal tunnel syndrome, tendonitis etc.

To join this discussion list send the following message:

To: listserv@itssrv1.ucsf.edu
Text: subscribe sorehand *firstname lastname*

Web archive of messages (and background information) available at:
<http://www.ucsf.edu/sorehand/>.

Online newsgroup

Though there is no newsgroup devoted to carpal tunnel syndrome, postings on this subject are regularly found in the <news://alt.support.chronic-pain> newsgroup.

Name of newsgroup: <news://alt.support.chronic-pain>

To view the Web archive of messages, go to <http://groups.google.com/> and enter the following: alt.support.chronic.pain

Suggested summary documents

The Arthritis Research Campaign has produced an online information booklet describing symptoms, causes and treatment, illustrated with line drawings. It is available at: <http://www.arc.org.uk/about_arth/booklets/6008/6008.htm>.

The American Medical Association hosts a patient information page, which also includes tips on prevention. It can be found at: <http://www.ama-assn.org/insight/spec_con/patient/pat059.htm>.

Cataracts

Support group
Royal National Institute for the Blind (RNIB)
224 Great Portland Street
London
W1N 6AA

Tel: 0845 766 9999 (Textphone users call via Typetalk 0800 51 51 52)
Fax: 020 7388 2034
E-mail: helpline@rnib.org.uk
Web page: <http://www.rnib.org.uk>

Online discussion list
Name of list: **Lowvis (Low Vision Discussion List)**

To join this discussion list send the following message:

To: listserv@maelstrom.stjohns.edu
Text: subscribe lowvis

Web archive of messages available at:
<http://maelstrom.stjohns.edu/archives/lowvis.html>

Online newsgroup
Name of newsgroup: <news://sci.med.vision>

To view the Web archive of messages, go to <http://groups.google.com/> and enter the following: sci.med.vision

Suggested summary documents
The RNIB have produced a guide called 'Understanding cataracts'. As well as describing causes and symptoms, it advises on what would happen during and after an operation. It can be found at: <http://www.rnib.org.uk/info/cataract.htm>. The RNIB also offer a related guide to 'Childhood cataracts', available at: <http://www.rnib.org.uk/info/childcat.htm>.

In its 'Information for Patients' series, the US National Eye Institute offers a guide to cataracts. This can be downloaded from: <http://www.nei.nih.gov/publications/cataracts.htm>.

Cerebral palsy

Support group
SCOPE
PO Box 833
Milton Keynes
Bucks
MK12 5NY

Tel: 0808 800 3333
Fax: 01908 321051
E-mail: cphelpline@scope.org.uk
Web page: <http://www.scope.org.uk/>

Online discussion list
Name of list: **C-PALSY**

Discussion list established for parents who have a child with cerebral palsy.

To join this discussion list send the following message:

To: listserv@maelstrom.stjohns.edu
Text: subscribe c-palsy

Web archive of messages available at:
<http://maelstrom.stjohns.edu/archives/c-palsy.html>

Online newsgroup
Name of newsgroup: <news://alt.support.cerebral-palsy>

To view the Web archive of messages, go to <http://groups.google.com/> and enter the following: alt.support.cerebral-palsy

Suggested summary documents
The US National Institute of Neurological Disorders and Stroke (NINDS) hosts an information page that describes the condition and discusses treatment and prognosis. It is available at:
<http://www.ninds.nih.gov/health_and_medical/disorders/cerebral_palsy.htm>.

The US charity March of Dimes provides a more detailed page at:
<http://www.modimes.org/HealthLibrary2/FactSheets/Cerebral_Palsy.htm>.

In the UK, SCOPE offers a range of online fact sheets on various topics related to cerebral palsy, available at: <http://www.scope.org.uk/action/factsheets/index.shtml>.

Cervical cancer

See also **Cancer.**

Support group
Women's Nationwide Cancer Control Campaign
Suna House
128–130 Curtain Road
London
EC2A 3AQ

Tel: 020 7729 4688
Fax: 020 7613 0771
E-mail: wnccc@dial.pipex.com
Web page: <http://www.wnccc.org.uk/>

A more general support group is CancerBACUP
Web page: <http://www.cancerbacup.org.uk>

Online discussion list
Name of list: **Cervical-cancer-L list**

To join this discussion list send the following message:

To: listserv@info.path.org
Text: subscribe cervical-cancer-l

Web archive of messages available at: <http://info.path.org/archives/cervical-cancer-l.html>

Online newsgroup
Name of newsgroup: <news://alt.support.cancer>

To view the Web archive of messages, go to <http://groups.google.com/> and enter the following: alt.support.cancer

Suggested summary documents
CancerBACUP provides an online brochure called 'Understanding cancer of the cervix' which explains how cervical cancer develops and discusses diagnosis and treatment. It can be viewed at:
<http://www.cancerbacup.org.uk/info/cervix.htm>.

The US Women's Cancer Network provides information about cervical cancer, including factors that increase or decrease likely risk. It is available at:
<http://www.wcn.org/cancer_info/cervical.htm>.

The American National Cancer Institute provides more detailed information at: <http://cancernet.nci.nih.gov/wyntk_pubs/cervix.htm>.

Chronic fatigue syndrome (CFS)

See also **Fibromyalgia.**

Support group
ME Association
4 Corringham Road
Stanford-le-Hope
Essex
SS17 0AH

Tel: 01375 642466
Fax: 01375 360256
E-mail: membership@meassociation.org.uk
Web page: <http://www.meassociation.org.uk/>

Online discussion list

Name of list: **Co-Cure** ('Cooperate and Communicate for a Cure'): chronic fatigue syndrome and fibromyalgia information exchange.

Co-cure was established in 1996 as an information exchange forum intended to host a small volume of high-quality information, with the aim of furthering efforts to find a cure for CFS and fibromyalgia.

To join this discussion list send the following message:
To: listserv@listserv.nodak.edu
Text: subscribe co-cure

Web archive of messages available at: <http://listserv.nodak.edu/archives/co-cure.html>

Co-cure Web site: <http://www.co-cure.org/>

Online newsgroups

Name of newsgroup: <news://alt.med.cfs>

A UK-focused group is: <news://uk.people.support.cfs-me>

To view the Web archives of messages, go to <http://groups.google.com/> and enter either: alt.med.cfs *or* uk.people.support.cfs-me

Suggested summary documents

The ME Association has produced a brochure called 'What about ME? Your questions answered' which explains the difference between the terms ME (myalgic encephalomyelitis), CFS (chronic fatigue syndrome) and PVFS (post viral fatigue syndrome). It also discusses symptoms and management. It can be found at: <http://www.meassociation.org.uk/wameyqa.htm>.

The House of Commons Library has produced a paper about the controversy surrounding CFS, available as paper no 98/107 at:
<http://www.parliament.uk/commons/lib/research/rp98/rp98.htm>

The US National Center for Infectious Diseases maintains a 'Chronic fatigue syndrome home page' at:
<http://www.cdc.gov/ncidod/diseases/cfs/cfshome.htm>.

Cirrhosis

Support group
British Liver Trust
Ransomes Europark
Ipswich
IP3 9QG

Tel: 01473 276326
Fax: 01473 276327
E-mail: info@britishlivertrust.org.uk
Web page: <http://www.britishlivertrust.org.uk/>

Online discussion list
Name of list: **HEPV-L**

This list is primarily for discussion of hepatitis, but includes cirrhosis.

To join send the following message:

To: listserv@maelstrom.stjohns.edu
Text: sub hepv-l *firstname lastname*

Web archive of messages available at:
<http://maelstrom.stjohns.edu/archives/hepv-l.html>

Online newsgroup
Name of newsgroup: <news://sci.med.diseases.hepatitis>

To view the Web archive of messages, go to <http://groups.google.com/> and enter the following: sci.med.diseases.hepatitis

Suggested summary documents
The British Liver Trust provides a very clear information leaflet, covering causes, symptoms, diagnosis and treatment, as well as the connection between cirrhosis and hepatitis. It is available at:
<http://www.britishlivertrust.org.uk/publications/cirrhosis.html>.

The American Gastroenterological Association has produced a useful overview of causes, symptoms, diagnosis and treatment. It is available at: <http://www.gastro.org/public/cirrhosis.html>.

The US National Digestive Diseases Information Clearinghouse provides a detailed online guide at: <http://www.niddk.nih.gov/health/digest/pubs/cirrhosi/cirrhosi.htm>.

Coeliac disease

Support group

The Coeliac Society
PO Box 220
High Wycombe
Bucks
HP11 2HY

Tel: 01494 437278
Fax: 01494 474349
E-mail: admin@coeliac.co.uk
Web page: <http://www.coeliac.co.uk/>

Online discussion list

Name of list: **CELIAC**

CELIAC is an open, unmoderated discussion list for those interested in coeliac disease (coeliac sprue), dermatitis herpetiformis, gluten intolerance, wheat allergy, and co-incident intolerances, such as casein or lactose intolerance.

To join this discussion list send the following message:

To: listserv@maelstrom.stjohns.edu
Text: subscribe celiac *firstname lastname*

Web archive of messages available at:
<http://maelstrom.stjohns.edu/archives/celiac.html>

The list has an associated Web site, offering more information about coeliac disease and gluten-free diet; available at: <http://www.enabling.org/ia/celiac/index.html>.

Online newsgroup

Name of newsgroup: <news://alt.support.celiac>

To view the Web archive of messages, go to <http://groups.google.com/> and enter the following: alt.support.celiac

Suggested summary documents

As part of a series of patient information leaflets, the Digestive Disorders Foundation provides an online leaflet describing coeliac disease. This includes a description of the investigations needed to determine gluten sensitivity. It can be found at:

<http://www.digestivedisorders.org.uk/leaflets/coeliac.html>.

The US National Digestive Diseases Information Clearinghouse also provides a clear and detailed online guide at:
<http://www.niddk.nih.gov/health/digest/pubs/celiac/index.htm>.

Colorectal cancer

See also **Cancer.**

Support groups

Colon Cancer Concern
9 Rickett Street
London
SW6 1RU

Tel: 020 7381 9711
E-mail: help@coloncancer.org.uk
Web page: <http://www.coloncancer.org.uk/>

Beating Bowel Cancer (formerly known as the Crocus Trust)
PO Box 360
Twickenham
Middx
TW1 1UN

Tel: 020 8892 5256
Fax: 020 8744 2266
E-mail: info@beatingbowelcancer.org
Web page: <http://www.bowelcancer.org/>

Online discussion list
Name of list: **COLON**

This list provides various kinds of support relating to colon cancer.

To join this discussion list send the following message:

To: listserv@listserv.acor.org
Text: subscribe colon

Web archive of messages available at:
<http://listserv.acor.org/archives/colon.html>

Online newsgroup
Name of newsgroup: <news://alt.support.cancer>

To view the Web archive of messages, go to <http://groups.google.com/> and enter the following: alt.support.cancer

Suggested summary documents

CancerBACUP has produced a booklet called 'Understanding cancer of the colon and rectum', which answers questions about diagnosis and treatment. It can be found at: <http://www.bacup.org.uk/info/colon.htm>.

The US National Cancer Institute also provides a useful overview, which includes an outline of risk factors and advice on reducing the risk. It is available at: <http://cancernet.nci.nih.gov/wyntk_pubs/colon.htm>.

Cot death

See **Sudden infant death syndrome (SIDS).**

Creutzfeldt–Jakob disease (CJD)

Support group
CJD Support Network
Birchwood
Heath Top
Ashley Heath
Market Drayton
Shropshire
TF9 4QR

Tel: 01630 673 973
Fax: 01630 673 993
E-mail: cjdnet@alzheimers.org.uk
Web page: <http://www.alzheimers.org.uk/cjd/index.html>
And also: <http://glaxocentre.merseyside.org/cjd1.html>

Online discussion list
Name of list: **CJD Voice**

CJD Voice provides support and information for people who have loved ones who have died or are dying of CJD.

To join this discussion list go to the Web site <http://www.cjdvoice.org> and follow the links to the discussion page.

Online newsgroup

Although at the time of writing there was no newsgroup that focuses exclusively on CJD, the subject has been discussed in a wide variety of groups, including: <news://misc.kids.health>.

Name of newsgroup: <news://misc.kids.health>

To view the Web archive of messages, go to <http://groups.google.com/> and enter the following: misc.kids.health

Suggested summary documents

The *British Medical Journal* (*BMJ*) has produced a Web page providing links to government statements and *BMJ* extracts on bovine spongiform encephalopathy (BSE) and Creutzfeldt–Jakob disease (CJD). It can be found at: <http://www.bmj.com/bse.htm>.

The homepage of the BSE Inquiry is at: <http://www.bse.org.uk/>.

The US National Institute of Neurological Disorders and Stroke has created a CJD fact sheet that describes the symptoms and diagnosis and discusses causes and means of transmission. It can be found at:
<http://www.ninds.nih.gov/health_and_medical/pubs/
creutzfeldt-jakob_disease_fact_sheet.htm>.

Crohn's disease

Support group

NACC (National Association for Colitis and Crohn's Disease)
4 Beaumont House
Sutton Road
St Albans
Hertfordshire
AL1 5HH

Tel (Helpline): 01727 844296
Fax: 01727 862550
E-mail: nacc@nacc.org.uk
Web page: <http://www.nacc.org.uk/>

Online discussion list

Name of list: **Crohns**

A forum for discussion of Crohn's disease, including advances in treatments and medications as well as general discussion on coping with it.

To join this discussion list send the following message:

To: crohns-subscribe@yahoogroups.com
Text: leave blank

Web archive of messages available at:
<http://groups.yahoo.com/group/Crohns>

Online newsgroup

Name of newsgroup: <news://alt.support.crohns-colitis>

To view the Web archive of messages, go to <http://groups.google.com/> and enter the following: alt.support.crohns-colitis

Suggested summary documents

The Digestive Disorders Foundation has produced a leaflet on 'Ulcerative colitis and Crohn's disease', explaining the similarities and describing symptoms, diagnosis and treatment. It is available at: <http://www.digestivedisorders.org.uk/leaflets/colitis.html>.

The Crohn's and Colitis Foundation of America provides 'basic facts' about the conditions, and other types of inflammatory bowel disease, available at: <http://www.ccfa.org/medcentral/library/basic/>.

Cystic fibrosis

Support group

Cystic Fibrosis Trust
11 London Road
Bromley
Kent
BR1 1BY

Tel: 020 8464 7211
Fax: 020 8313 0472
E-mail: enquiries@cftrust.org.uk
Web page: <http://www.cftrust.org.uk/>

Online discussion list

Name of list: **CYSTIC-L**

CYSTIC-L is an e-mail support-group for people with cystic fibrosis (CF) and their friends, families, and healthcare providers. It includes both 'casual banter about the varied impact that CF has on our lives, as well as technical and medical information exchanges'. An extensive FAQ (frequently asked questions), which contains much CF information, and references to other CF resources is available to subscribers.

To join this discussion list send the following message:

To: listserv@home.ease.lsoft.com
Text: subscribe cystic-l

Web archive of messages available at:
<http://home.ease.lsoft.com/archives/cystic-l.html>

Online newsgroup

At the time of writing, there was no newsgroup specifically related to cystic fibrosis. However, the subject has been discussed in a variety of groups, including: <news://misc.kids.health>.

Name of newsgroup: <news://misc.kids.health>

To view the Web archive of messages, go to <http://groups.google.com/> and enter the following: misc.kids.health

Suggested summary documents

The Cystic Fibrosis Resource Centre (produced by Solvay Healthcare Ltd) is a useful source of information for cystic fibrosis patients, parents, doctors and other carers <http://www.cysticfibrosis.co.uk/>. It includes news items, information on medical research and available treatments, and links to other sites. A free e-mail newsletter is available.

The US Cystic Fibrosis Foundation also maintains a fact sheet about the condition, available at: <http://www.cff.org/facts.htm>.

Cystitis (interstitial)

Support group
Interstitial Cystitis Support Group
76 High Street
Stony Stratford
Bucks
MK11 1AH

Tel or Fax: 01908 569169
E-mail: info@interstitialcystitis.co.uk
Web page: <http://www.interstitialcystitis.co.uk/>

Online discussion list

Name of list: **ICSUPPORT**

The Interstitial Cystitis Support e-mail list is intended for sharing 'remedies, medical procedures, and anything related to IC, including how it has changed your life and how you have been dealing with the changes. You can come to vent and share, seek support or give support.'

To join this discussion list send the following message:

To: listserv@maelstrom.stjohns.edu
Subject: icsupport
Text: subscribe icsupport *firstname lastname*

Web archive of messages available at:
<http://maelstrom.stjohns.edu/archives/icsupport.html>

Online newsgroup

Name of newsgroup: <news://alt.support.inter-cystitis>

To view the Web archive of messages, go to <http://groups.google.com/> and enter the following: alt.support.inter-cystitis

Suggested summary documents

The US National Institute of Diabetes and Digestive and Kidney Diseases provides a useful overview of this condition, covering symptoms, diagnosis and treatment. It can be found at:
<http://www.niddk.nih.gov/health/urolog/pubs/cystitis/cystitis.htm#1>.

More detailed information can be found on the Web site of the US Interstitial Cystitis Association, particularly in the sections called 'What is IC', found at <http://www.ichelp.org/WhatIsIC/welcome.html>, and 'Treatment options' at <http://www.ichelp.org/TreatmentAndSelfHelp/welcome.html>.

Deafness

Support group

Royal National Institute for Deaf People (RNID)
19–23 Featherstone Street
London

EC1Y 8SL

Tel: 0808 808 0123
Fax: 020 7296 8199
E-mail: helpline@rnid.org.uk
Web page: <http://www.rnid.org.uk/>

Online discussion list

Name of list: **Deaf-L**

For the discussion of questions, topics, and concerns related to deafness.

To join this discussion list send the following message:

To: listserv@siu.edu
Text: subscribe deaf-l

Online newsgroups

Name of newsgroup: <news://bit.listserv.deaf-l>

There is also a UK-based group: <news://uk.people.deaf>

To view the Web archives of messages, go to <http://groups.google.com/>
and enter either: bit.listserv.deaf-l *or* uk.people.deaf

Suggested summary documents

The RNID has produced a wide range of informative leaflets about aspects of
deafness and hearing loss, available from:
<http://www.rnid.org.uk/html/info_factsheets.htm>.

The British Deaf Association is developing a Web site at
<http://www.britishdeafassociation.org.uk/> which is designed to reflect all
aspects of deaf culture.

Contact A Family, a UK charity, has produced a fact sheet on deafness, which
explains different types of deafness and lists a range of support
organisations. It can be found at:
<http://www.cafamily.org.uk/Direct/d18.html>.

Dementia

See **Alzheimer's disease.**

Depression

See also **Seasonal Affective Disorder (SAD).**

Support groups
Depression Alliance
35 Westminster Bridge Road
London
SE1 7JB

Tel: 020 7633 0557
Fax: 020 7633 0559
E-mail: hq@depressionalliance.org
Web page: <http://www.depressionalliance.org/>

Mind
Granta House
15–19 Broadway
Stratford
London
E15 4BQ

Tel: 020 8522 1728
Fax: 020 8522 1725
E-mail: contact@mind.org.uk
Web page: <http://www.mind.org.uk/>

Online discussion list
Name of list: **DAtalk**

This list is intended for users to share experiences and coping strategies with others in similar situations. The service is available only to Depression Alliance members. For more information, e-mail the list owner at: datalk-owner@egroups.com

Online newsgroups
Name of newsgroup: <news://alt.support.depression>

There is also a UK-based group: <news://uk.people.support.depression>

To view the Web archives of messages, go to <http://groups.google.com/> and enter either: alt.support.depression *or* uk.people.support.depression

Suggested summary documents

The Mental Health Foundation has published a booklet called 'All about depression' which examines different kinds of depression, causes, ways of coping, and a list of sources of further information. It is available at: <http://www.mentalhealth.org.uk/bkdepress.htm>.

NHS Direct Online had a theme month for depression, with a Web site at <http://cebmh.warne.ox.ac.uk/cebmh/nelmh/depression/>.

The National Institute of Mental Health (USA) has produced a range of clear and informative brochures on aspects of depression; a list can be found at: <http://www.nimh.nih.gov/publicat/depressionmenu.cfm>.

Dermatitis

See **Acne** and **Eczema**

Diabetes

Support group

Diabetes UK (Formerly British Diabetic Association)
10 Queen Anne Street
London
W1G 9LH

Tel: 020 7323 1531
Fax: 020 7637 3644
E-mail: info@diabetes.org.uk
Web page: <http://www.diabetes.org.uk/>

Online discussion list
Name of list: **DIABETES-EHLB**

Online diabetes discussion list for people with diabetes.

To join this discussion list send the following message:

To: listserv@shrsys.hslc.org
Text: subscribe diabetes-ehlb

Web archive of messages available at: <http://www.hslc.org/archives/diabetes-ehlb.html>

Online newsgroup

Name of newsgroup: <news://alt.support.diabetes>

To view the Web archive of messages, go to <http://groups.google.com/> and enter the following: alt.support.diabetes

Suggested summary documents

The US National Institute of Diabetes and Digestive and Kidney Diseases publishes detailed information in the form of a range of online publications, which are listed at: <http://www.niddk.nih.gov/health/diabetes/diabetes.htm>. They include a useful overview which describes different types of diabetes and discusses management of the condition: <http://www.niddk.nih.gov/health/diabetes/pubs/dmover/dmover.htm>.

The International Diabetes Institute has an informative Web site at <http://www.diabetes.com.au/home.htm>. Although it is based in Australia and has an Australian emphasis, it is aimed at a global community.

Down's syndrome

Support group

Down's Syndrome Association
153–155 Mitcham Road
London
SW17 9PG

Tel: 020 8682 4001
Fax: 020 8682 4012
E-mail: info@downs-syndrome.org.uk
Web page: <http://www.dsa-uk.com/>

Online discussion list

Name of list: **DOWN-SYN**

This list is for discussion of Down's syndrome, and is open to parents, siblings, friends, doctors, teachers as well as people with Down's syndrome.

To join this discussion list send the following message:

To: listserv@listserv.nodak.edu
Text: subscribe down-syn

Web archive of messages available at:

<http://listserv.nodak.edu/archives/down-syn.html>

(*see also:* The Down Syndrome Information Network, below)

Online newsgroup

Name of newsgroup: <news://bit.listserv.down-syn>

To view the Web archive of messages, go to <http://groups.google.com/> and enter the following: bit.listserv.down-syn

Suggested summary documents

The Down Syndrome Information Network offers a range of information resources and online services, including a range of e-mail discussion lists. It aims to provide information and services to the international Down's syndrome community, including families, carers, professionals and researchers. The home page is at: <http://www.down-syndrome.net/>. (It is currently funded by The Down Syndrome Educational Trust, a UK registered charity.)

The US National Down Syndrome Society (NDSS) has a Web page containing general information about Down's syndrome. Particular features include lists of 'questions and answers', 'myths and truths', and a list of recommendations for further reading. It is available at:
<http://www.ndss.org/aboutds/aboutds.html#parent>.

The March of Dimes Birth Defects Foundation, based in the US, has produced a Down's syndrome fact sheet, available at:
<http://www.modimes.org/HealthLibrary2/FactSheets/Down_syndrome.htm>.

Drug abuse

Support group

DrugScope
Waterbridge House
32–36 Loman Street
London SE1 0EE

Tel: 0207 928 1211
Fax: 0207 928 1771
E-mail: services@drugscope.org.uk
Web page: <http://www.drugscope.org.uk/>

Online discussion list

Yahoo! Groups hosts a range of discussion groups in the section:
Top ◊ Health & Wellness ◊ Support ◊ Addiction and Recovery ◊ Drugs.

A list can be found at: <http://dir.groups.yahoo.com/dir/1600061541>. At the time of writing, there were 39 different lists covering many aspects of drug abuse. For example:

Name of list: **narecovery**

Addicts working together to recover from the disease of addiction using the 12 steps of Narcotics Anonymous.

To join this discussion list send a blank e-mail:

To: narecovery-subscribe@yahoogroups.com
Text: leave blank

Web archive of messages: for members only.

Online newsgroup

Name of newsgroup: <news://alt.recovery>

To view the Web archive of messages, go to <http://groups.google.com/> and enter the following: alt.recovery

Suggested summary documents

Health Promotion England has produced a Web site called 'Trashed' <http://www.trashed.co.uk/> which provides clear and well-structured information on a range of drugs. For each drug listed the site details its legal status, the effects it has on the body, and the dangers it poses.

DrugScope runs a Web service called LOCATE <http://www.locatenet.org.uk/>, aimed at people providing drug education and prevention for young people, their parents and carers. It collects and disseminates information on organisations and their drug education and prevention activities.

The US National Institute on Drug Addiction has produced a range of information on drug abuse and addiction, including a set of guides on the health effects of specific drugs. The guides are listed at: <http://www.drugabuse.gov/Infofax/Infofaxindex.html>.

Dyslexia

Support group

British Dyslexia Association
98 London Road
Reading
Berks
RG1 5AU

Tel: 0118 966 8271
Fax: 0118 935 1927
E-mail: info@dyslexiahelp-bda.demon.co.uk
Web page: <http://www.bda-dyslexia.org.uk/>

Online discussion list

Name of list: **Dyslexia**

Discussion list by, and for, dyslexic people.

To join this discussion list send the following message:

To: jiscmail@jiscmail.ac.uk
Text: join dyslexia *firstname lastname*

Web archive of messages available at:
<http://www.jiscmail.ac.uk/lists/dyslexia.html>

Online newsgroup

Name of newsgroup: <news://alt.support.dyslexia>

To view the Web archive of messages, go to <http://groups.google.com/> and enter the following: alt.support.dyslexia

Suggested summary documents

The Dyslexia Institute provides a range of information on its Web site at <http://www.dyslexia-inst.org.uk/infomenu.htm>, including advice for parents and teachers on how to recognise it.

The National Information Center for Children and Youth with Disabilities has produced a briefing paper on the more general subject of reading and learning disabilities. It can be found at:
<http://www.nichcy.org/pubs/factshe/fs17txt.htm>.

Eating disorders

See **Anorexia nervosa** and **Bulimia.**

Eczema

Support group

The National Eczema Society
Hill House
Highgate Hill
London
N19 5NA

Tel: 0870 241 3604
Fax: 020 7281 6395
E-mail: eczema@nes.comu-netcom
Web page: <http://www.eczema.org/>

Online discussion list

Name of list: **Eczema**

The list aims to allow people with eczema to share their experiences of living with and managing eczema. It is also open to people such as parents of children with eczema and people with a professional interest in eczema.

To join this discussion list send the following message:

To: listserv@maelstrom.stjohns.edu
Text: subscribe eczema

Web archive of messages available at:
<http://maelstrom.stjohns.edu/archives/eczema.html>

Online newsgroup

Name of newsgroup: <news://alt.support.skin-diseases>

To view the Web archive of messages, go to <http://groups.google.com/> and enter the following: alt.support.skin-diseases

Suggested summary documents

The National Eczema Society has produced a Web page of 'Frequently asked questions' (FAQs) about eczema, available at: <http://www.eczema.org/faqfile.htm>.

The American Academy of Dermatology provides information on eczema and atopic dermatitis on its Web site at <http://www.aad.org/pamphlets/eczema.html>, as well as a wide variety of information aimed at the general public: <http://www.aad.org/patient_intro.html>.

The US National Institute of Arthritis and Musculoskeletal and Skin Diseases has produced a handout on atopic dermatitis, which describes the disease and its symptoms. It contains information about diagnosis and treatment as well as current research efforts. It can be found at: <http://www.nih.gov/niams/healthinfo/dermatitis/atophandout_breaks.html>.

The US National Eczema Association has produced a Web document called 'The Basics' which offers advice on how to go about making treatment decisions. It can be found at: <http://www.eczema-assn.org/the_basics.html>. More generally, the American Academy of Family Physicians offers tips on how to care for your skin at: <http://familydoctor.org/handouts/176.html>.

Emphysema

Support group
Breathe Easy Club
British Lung Foundation
78 Hatton Garden
London
EC1N 8LD

Tel: 020 7831 5831
Fax: 020 7831 5832
E-mail: breatheasy@britishlungfoundation.com
Web page: <http://www.lunguk.org/breathe/index.html>

Information about regional offices can be found at: <http://www.lunguk.org/area/index.html>

Online discussion list
Name of list: **COPD/Emphysema Online Support Mailing List**

The mailing list is intended to be a means by which people can share information and support concerning this disease. 'In this way it contributes to the longevity and quality of life.'

To join this discussion list send the following message:

To: listserv@home.ease.lsoft.com
Text: subscribe copd

Web archive of messages available at:
<http://home.ease.lsoft.com/archives/copd.html>

Online newsgroup

Although there is no newsgroup that focuses exclusively on emphysema, the topic is discussed in the asthma newsgroup.

Name of newsgroup: <news://alt.support.asthma>

To view the Web archive of messages, go to <http://groups.google.com/> and enter the following: alt.support.asthma

Suggested summary documents

The US National Emphysema Foundation has produced a fact sheet on chronic obstructive pulmonary disease, which covers emphysema. As well as causes, symptoms and treatment, it includes information on pulmonary function tests. It can be found at:
<http://www.emphysemafoundation.org/copdcbro.htm>.

The US National Heart, Lung, and Blood Institute has produced a useful overview of chronic obstructive pulmonary disease. The online brochure is available at:
<http://www.nhlbi.nih.gov/health/public/lung/other/copd/copd_toc.htm>.

Encephalitis

Support group

Encephalitis Support Group
44a Market Place
Malton
North Yorkshire
YO17 7LW

Tel/Fax: 01653 699 599
E-mail: encephalitissupportgroup@compuserve.com
Web page: <http://glaxocentre.merseyside.org/1enceph.html>

Online discussion list

Name of list: **Encephalitis Support Group Mailing List**

This is an open mailing list intended to facilitate contact between people affected by encephalitis.

To join this discussion list send the following message:

To: majordomo@connect.org.uk
Text: subscribe esg@connect.org.uk

Online newsgroup

Though there is no newsgroup that focuses exclusively on encephalitis, the topic is discussed in the Lyme disease newsgroup:

Name of newsgroup: <news://sci.med.diseases.lyme>

To view the Web archive of messages, go to <http://groups.google.com/> and enter the following: sci.med.disease.lyme

Suggested summary documents

The Encephalitis Support Group has extensive information on its Web site, including an overview called 'What is encephalitis?' <http://glaxocentre.merseyside.org/1enceph.htm>.

The US National Institute of Neurological Disorders and Stroke has produced a 'Meningitis and Encephalitis information page' which offers a brief overview of this condition <http://www.ninds.nih.gov/health_and_medical/disorders/encmenin_doc.htm>.

Endometriosis

Support groups

National Endometriosis Society
Suite 50
Westminster Palace Gardens
1–7 Artillery Row
London
SW1P 1RL

Tel: 020 7222 2776
Fax: 020 7222 2786
E-mail: endoinfo@compuserve.com
Web page: <http://www.endo.org.uk>

Online discussion list

Yahoo! Groups hosts 26 discussion lists on aspects of endometriosis. A list of them can be viewed at:

<http://dir.groups.yahoo.com/dir/Health_Wellness/Support/Illnesses/Endometriosis>.

The list with the largest membership is: **erc (Endometriosis Research Center)**.

The list is intended for women and girls to communicate, share experiences and learn about endometriosis and related topics.

For more information, see <http://groups.yahoo.com/group/erc> and <http://www.endocenter.org/>.

To join this discussion list, send a blank e-mail

To: erc-subscribe@yahoogroups.com
Text: leave blank

Online newsgroup
Name of newsgroup: <news://alt.support.endometriosis>

To view the Web archive of messages, go to <http://groups.google.com/> and enter the following: alt.support.endometriosis

Suggested summary documents
Detailed information on endometriosis is available on the Women's Health Information Web site <http://www.womens-health.co.uk/endo.htm>. The document explains causes, diagnosis and treatment options, and includes a reference list for further reading.

The US National Institute of Child health and Human Development has produced a Web page called 'Facts about endometriosis', which looks at causes, symptoms, diagnosis and treatment, as well as links to fertility problems. It can be found at:
<http://www.nichd.nih.gov/publications/pubs/endomet.htm>.

Finally, the Endometriosis Research Center provides a range of useful information on its Web site at: <http://www.endocenter.org/>.

Enuresis

Support group
Enuresis Resource and Information Centre (ERIC)
34 Old School House
Britannia Road
Kingswood
Bristol
BS15 2DB

Tel: 0117 960 3060
Fax: 0117 960 0401
E-mail: info@eric.org.uk
Web page: <http://www.enuresis.org.uk/main.html>
And also: <http://www.eric.org.uk/> (registration necessary)

Online discussion list
Name of list: **Enuresis Support and Information Group (ESIG)**

To join this discussion list send the following message:

To: listserv@maelstrom.stjohns.edu
Text: subscribe enuresis

Web archive of messages available at:
<http://maelstrom.stjohns.edu/archives/enuresis.html>

Online newsgroup
Name of newsgroup: <news://misc.kids>

This group covers a very broad range of subjects, but has included some discussion of bedwetting in children.

To view the Web archive of messages, go to <http://groups.google.com/> and enter the following: misc.kids

Suggested summary documents
The Enuresis Resource and Information Centre produces information for parents on how best to manage a child who suffers from this condition, available at: <http://www.enuresis.org.uk/parents.html>. The Mayo Clinic provides an overview called 'Bedwetting: strategies for solution', also aimed at parents. It can be found at:
<http://www.mayohealth.org/mayo/9601/htm/bedwet.htm>.

Information about bedwetting aimed at children can be found on the US-based Kidshealth site at:
<http://kidshealth.org/kid/health_problems/enuresis.html>.

Epilepsy

Support group
British Epilepsy Association
New Anstey House
Gateway Drive
Yeadon
Leeds
West Yorkshire
LS19 7XY

Tel: 0808 800 5050
Fax: 0113 391 0300
E-mail: epilepsy@bea.org.uk
Web page: <http://www.epilepsy.org.uk/>

Online discussion list
Name of list: **Epilepsy-L**

This is an e-mail support group for people with epilepsy (often referred to as 'PwEs' on this list), and for their friends, families, doctors, etc – 'anyone who cares for them and about them'.

To join this discussion list send the following message:

To: listserv@home.ease.lsoft.com
Text: subscribe epilepsy-l

Web archive of messages available at:
<http://home.ease.lsoft.com/archives/epilepsy-l.html>

Online newsgroup
Name of newsgroup: <news://alt.support.epilepsy>

There is also a UK-based group:

Name of newsgroup: <news://uk.people.support.epilepsy>

To view the Web archive of messages, go to <http://groups.google.com/> and enter either: alt.support.epilepsy *or* uk.people.support.epilepsy

Suggested summary documents

The National Society for Epilepsy has produced an informative Web page describing the different types of epilepsy, causes, diagnosis and treatment options. It includes a booklist of recommended reading. It is available at: <http://www.epilepsynse.org.uk/pages/info/leaflets/explaini.html>.

The US National Institute of Neurological Disorders and Stroke has produced a Web page called 'Seizures and epilepsy: hope through research'. This includes detailed information about causes, diagnosis, prevention and treatment of epilepsy. It can be found at: <http://www.ninds.nih.gov/health_and_medical/pubs/seizures_and_ epilepsy_htr.htm>.

Fibromyalgia

See also **Chronic Fatigue Syndrome (CFS).**

Support group

Fibromyalgia Association UK
PO Box 206
Stourbridge
DY9 8YL

Tel: 01384 820052
Fax: 01384 869467
E-mail: fms@cableinet.co.uk
Web page: <http://www.ukfibromyalgia.com/>

Fibromyalgia Support Northern Ireland has a Web site at <http://www.fmsni.freeserve.co.uk/>.

Online discussion list

Name of list: **Co-Cure**

Co-Cure has been established with the goal of 'furthering co-operative efforts towards finding the cure for chronic fatigue syndrome (CFS) and the related fibromyalgia (FM) through the open distribution and exchange of information between the medical/clinical, political, and patient groups, as well as other organizations/institutions'.

To join this discussion list send the following message:

To: listserv@listserv.nodak.edu
Text: subscribe co-cure

Web archive of messages available at: <http://listserv.nodak.edu/archives/co-cure.html>

Online newsgroup
Name of newsgroup: <news://alt.med.fibromyalgia>

To view the Web archive of messages, go to <http://groups.google.com/> and enter the following: alt.med.fibromyalgia

Suggested summary documents
The US National Institute of Arthritis and Musculoskeletal and Skin Diseases has produced a Web page of 'Questions and answers about fibromyalgia', which describes the condition and looks at causes, symptoms and treatment. It can be found at: <http://www.nih.gov/niams/healthinfo/fibrofs.htm>.

The Mayo Clinic provides a resource called 'Fibromyalgia: coping with the pain'. It provides links to pages about fibromyalgia and sleep, and about managing pain. It is available at:
<http://www.mayohealth.org/mayo/9710/htm/fibromya.htm>.

The American Academy of Family Physicians has produced a brief document on fibromyalgia and exercise, available at:
<http://www.familydoctor.org/handouts/061.html>.

Food allergy

Support group
Anaphylaxis Campaign
PO Box 149
Fleet
Hampshire
GU13 0FA

Tel: 01252 542029
Fax: 01252 377140
E-mail: n/a
Web page: <http://www.anaphylaxis.org.uk/>

Online discussion lists

Yahoo! Groups hosts at least 14 e-mail lists on food allergies – to see a list of them, go to: <http://dir.groups.yahoo.com/dir/1600061601>. A new discussion list, formed in January 2001, is described below:

Name of list: **The Food Allergy Kitchen**

An allergen-free recipe exchange. As recipes are posted, they are organised into categories for use like a cookbook. Messages posted are limited to recipes, questions about posted recipes (such as how to use substitutes), recipe requests, ingredient questions, or related food issues.

To join this discussion list send the following message:

To: foodallergykitchen-subscribe@yahoogroups.com
Text: leave blank

Web archive of messages: for members only.

More information available at: <http://groups.yahoo.com/group/FOODALLERGYKITCHEN>

Online newsgroup

Name of newsgroup: <news:alt.support.food-allergies>

To view the Web archive of messages, go to <http://groups.google.com/> and enter the following: alt.support.food-allergies

Suggested summary documents

The US National Institute of Allergy and Infectious Diseases (NIAID) has produced a guide called 'Food allergy and intolerances'. As well as discussing diagnosis and treatment, it explains some of the controversies surrounding food allergies.
<http://www.niaid.nih.gov/factsheets/food.htm>.

The US Food and Drug Administration provide an overview called 'Food allergies: rare but risky'. It explains the difference between an allergy and an intolerance, and looks at problems associated with some specific food additives. It can be viewed at: <http://vm.cfsan.fda.gov/~dms/wh-alrg1.html>.

Allergenica is an American Web site specialising in information about allergies. It has a section devoted to food allergies at:
<http://www.allergenica.com/Food.htm>.

Gallstones

Support group

British Liver Trust
Central House
Central Avenue
Ransomes Europark
Ipswich
Suffolk
IP3 9QG

Tel: 0808 800 1000
Fax: 01473 276327
E-mail: info@britishlivertrust.org.uk
Web page: <http://www.britishlivertrust.org.uk/>

Online discussion list

Name of list: **Gallstones**

A list for people to share information on cleansing gallstones from the liver and the gallbladder.

To join this discussion list send the following message:

To: gallstones-subscribe@yahoogroups.com
Text: leave blank

More information is available at: <http://groups.yahoo.com/group/gallstones>

Web archive of messages: for members only.

Online newsgroup

There is not a group specifically for gallstones, but they are occasionally discussed in the hepatitis newsgroup.

Name of newsgroup: <news://sci.med.diseases.hepatitis>

To view the Web archive of messages, go to <http://groups.google.com/> and enter the following: sci.med.diseases.hepatitis

Suggested summary documents

The British Liver Trust has produced an information leaflet on gallstones. It includes information on symptoms, tests and treatment, and can be found at:

<http://www.britishlivertrust.org.uk/publications/gallstones.html>.

The US National Institute of Diabetes and Digestive and Kidney Diseases (NIDDK) has produced a useful overview, which covers causes, symptoms, diagnosis and treatment of gallstones. It can be found at:
<http://www.niddk.nih.gov/health/digest/pubs/gallstns/gallstns.htm>.

They have also produced a related publication called 'Dieting and gallstones', available at:
<http://www.niddk.nih.gov/health/nutrit/pubs/dietgall.htm>.

Genetic disorders

Support group
Genetic Interest Group (GIG)
Unit 4d
Leroy House
436 Essex Road
London
N1 3QP

Tel: 020 7430 0090
Fax: 020 7359 1447
E-mail: post@gig.org.uk
Web page: <http://www.gig.org.uk/>

Online discussion list
Name of list: **gendisease-j**

A discussion list for individuals concerned with several specific inherited disorders. The list's subscribers include professionals, patients, researchers, religious leaders, students, parents, friends and others.

To join this discussion list send the following message:

To: listserv@maelstrom.stjohns.edu
Text: subscribe gendisease-j

Web archive of messages available at:
<http://maelstrom.stjohns.edu/archives/gendisease-j.html>

Further information about the list can be found at:
<http://www.gaucherdisease.org/list.htm>

Yahoo! Groups hosts nearly 100 discussion lists on genetic disorders, many of which focus on specific disorders. To see a list of them, go to:
<http://dir.groups.yahoo.com/dir/1600094714>.

Online newsgroups

Though there is no newsgroup devoted exclusively to genetic disorders the topic (sometimes referred to as 'chromosomal abnormalities') has been discussed in various groups – in particular <news://misc.kids.info> and <news://misc.kids.pregnancy>.

To view the Web archives of messages, go to <http://groups.google.com/> and enter either: misc.kids.info *or* misc.kids.pregnancy

Suggested summary documents

Contact a Family <http://www.cafamily.org.uk> is a UK charity providing support, advice and information to individuals and the parents of children with medical conditions (including unusual and rare conditions). An extremely useful feature of its Web site is the 'CaF Directory of Specific Conditions and Rare Disorders', available at: <http://www.cafamily.org.uk/dirworks.html>.

The Web site of the Public Health Genetics Unit <http://www.medinfo.cam.ac.uk/phgu/> provides news and information about advances in genetics and their impact on public health and the prevention of disease.

Glaucoma

Support group

International Glaucoma Association
108c Warner Road
Camberwell
London
SE5 9HQ

Tel: 020 7737 3265
Fax: 020 7346 5929
E-mail: info@iga.org.uk
Web page: <http://www.iga.org.uk/home.htm>

Online discussion list

Name of list: **Glaucoma mailing list**

This list aims to provide a safe atmosphere for glaucoma patients and medical professionals to come together for support and the discussion of glaucoma.

To join this discussion list send the following message:

To: glaucoma-subscribe@yahoogroups.com
Text: leave blank

Web archive of messages available at: <http://groups.yahoo.com/group/glaucoma>

Information page at:
<http://www.geocities.com/HotSprings/Resort/3929/listinfo.html>

Online newsgroup
Name of newsgroup: <news://alt.support.glaucoma>

To view the Web archive of messages, go to <http://groups.google.com/> and enter the following: alt.support.glaucoma

Suggested summary documents
The RNIB provides an overview on its Web site at <http://www.rnib.org.uk/info/glaucoma.htm>. 'Understanding glaucoma' includes details about different types of glaucoma, who is at risk, the symptoms and treatment. Contacts for further help and information are provided.

The US National Eye Institute provides a clear and informative pamphlet called 'Glaucoma: information for patients'. It includes a link to another pamphlet called 'Tips for talking to your doctor'. It can be found at: <http://www.nei.nih.gov/publications/glauc-pat.htm>.

Growth disorders

Support group
Restricted Growth Association
PO Box 4744
Dorchester
Dorset
DT2 9FA

Tel: 01308 898445
Fax: n/a
E-mail: rga1@talk21.com
Web page: <http://www.rgaonline.org.uk/>

Online discussion lists
Name of list: **HGF-PEDS**

This list is for people who have a child with a growth or growth-related disorder, and for people who are interested in human growth and/or growth disorders. The list exists to provide a forum to exchange ideas, information, news, comments, concerns, fears related to growth and growth disorders in children.

To join this discussion list send the following message:

To: listserv@home.ease.lsoft.com
Text: sub hgf-peds *firstname lastname*

More information is available at:
<http://www.familyvillage.wisc.edu/lists/hgf-peds.html>.

Name of list: HGF-ADULTS

This list, also created by the Human Growth Foundation, is for people who have adult growth hormone deficiency; and for people who are interested in adult growth hormone replacement therapy.

To join this discussion list send the following message:

To: listserv@home.ease.lsoft.com
Text: sub hgf-adults *firstname lastname*

More information is available at: <http://www.familyvillage.wisc.edu/lists/hgf-adults.html>.

Online newsgroups

Postings about growth disorders – especially achondroplasia – appear in a number of groups, identified below:

Name of newsgroup: <news://alt.support.short>
Name of newsgroups: <news://misc.handicap>

To view the Web archive of messages, go to <http://groups.google.com/> and enter either alt.support.short or misc.handicap

Suggested summary documents

The MAGIC (Major Aspects of Growth in Children) Foundation in the US has produced a number of 'informational brochures' covering topics such as 'The transition from child to adult growth hormone therapy' <http://www.magic-foundation.org/transition.html> and 'Underlying conditions of growth abnormalities' <http://www.magicfoundation.org/under.html> as well as more specific documents on identified conditions such as Turner's syndrome <http://www.magicfoundation.org/turners.html> and McCune-Albright syndrome <http://www.magicfoundation.org/mas.html>.

In the UK both the Child Growth Foundation <http://www.cgf.org.uk/info.html> and the Restricted Growth Association <http://www.rgaonline.org.uk/> have useful information on their sites, though some of this restricted to members.

For information on ongoing clinical trials both the US National Institutes of Health Clinical Trials site <http://clinicaltrails.gov> and CenterWatch <http://www.centerwatch.com/> provide up-to-date information. Note, however, that both these services are aimed at US consumers.

Gulf War syndrome

Support groups
Gulf Veterans' Medical Assessment Programme
The Baird Health Centre, Gassiot House, St Thomas' Hospital
Lambeth Palace Road, London SE1 7EH

Tel: 0800 169 5401
Fax: 020 7202 8327
Web page: <http://www.mod.uk/index.php3?page=971>

Veterans' Advice Line (run by Ministry of Defence): 08456 02 03 02 (Local Rate Call)

Online discussion lists
Two discussion lists are sponsored by the Gulf War Veteran Resource Pages Web Site <http://www.gulfweb.org/>

Name of list: **GWVM - Gulf War Veterans Mailing List**

The GWVM mailing list is intended to be used only for distributing 'hard' information that is directly related to Gulf War veterans' illnesses, and is not a public discussion forum. Debates and discussion of any type should be conducted on **Gulf-Chat** (see below).

To join this discussion list send the following message:

To: majordomo@structured.net
Text: subscribe gwvm *your e-mail address*

Web archive of messages available at:
<http://groups.yahoo.com/group/gwvm>

Name of list: **Gulf-Chat**

This list is provided for general Gulf War and veteran chat.

To join this discussion list send the following message:

To: majordomo@structured.net
Text: subscribe gulf-chat *your e-mail address*

Web archive of messages available at: <http://groups.yahoo.com/group/gulf-chat>

Online newsgroup

There is no group specifically for GWS, but there is a group for chronic fatigue syndrome <news://alt.med.cfs> which may be of interest.

To view the Web archive of messages, go to <http://groups.google.com/> and enter the following: alt.med.cfs

Suggested summary documents

GulfLink is an American site, produced by the American Department of Defense. As well as medical information, it includes news items and case narratives <http://www.gulflink.osd.mil/>.

The Official UK Ministry of Defence Web site devoted to Gulf Veterans' Illnesses can be found at <http://www.mod.uk/index.php3?page=955>. The site is provided to help Gulf veterans, and others interested in this issue, and to find out what the MOD is doing to help Gulf veterans.

Haemophilia

Support group

Haemophilia Society
Chesterfield House
385 Euston Road
London
NW1 3AU

Tel: 0800 018 6068
Fax: 020 7387 8220
E-mail: info@haemophilia.org.uk
Web page: <http://www.haemophilia.org.uk/>

Online discussion list

Name of list: **Hemophilia Support**

This discussion list is intended for both emotional support and sharing

medical information for people living with haemophilia. Further information about the list is available at:
<http://www.web-depot.com/hemophilia/hemophilia-support.info>.

To join this discussion list send the following message:

To: hemophilia-support-approval@web-depot.com
Text: subscribe hemophilia-support

Online newsgroup
Name of newsgroup: <news://alt.support.hemophilia>

To view the Web archive of messages, go to <http://groups.google.com/> and enter the following: alt.support.hemophilia

Suggested summary documents
The Haemophilia Society has produced a very clear 'Introduction to haemophilia'. It covers diagnosis, inheritance, treatment, and complications <http://www.haemophilia.org.uk/intromenu.html>.

The Oxford Haemophilia Centre offers a short article 'intended for those with no previous knowledge about haemophilia'. 'Haemophilia: some basic facts' is available at: <http://www.medicine.ox.ac.uk/ohc/basics.htm>.

The World Federation of Hemophilia has produced a very detailed Web page of 'frequently asked questions' (with answers). It includes both general guides and information about a range of very specific topics such as dental care or gene therapy. It can be found at:
<http://www.wfh.org/InformationAboutHemophilia/faq.htm>.

Hayfever

Support group
British Allergy Foundation
Deepdene House
30 Bellegrove Road
Welling
Kent
DA16 3PY

Tel: 020 8303 8583
Fax: 020 7601 8444
E-mail: allergybaf@compuserve.com
Web page: <http://www.allergyfoundation.com/>

Online discussion list

Name of list: **Allergy**

This list discusses all types of human allergies, including influence on health and lifestyles, treatments for allergies from the consumer perspective and experience, and self-help.

To join this discussion list send the following message:

To: listserv@listserv.uark.edu
Text: subscribe allergy *firstname lastname*

Web archive of messages available at: <http://www.immune.com/allergy>

Online newsgroup

Name of newsgroup: <news://alt.med.allergy>

To view the Web archive of messages, go to <http://groups.google.com/> and enter the following: alt.med.allergy

Suggested summary documents

The American Lung Association has produced a page called 'Facts about hayfever' that discusses causes, symptoms and control <http://www.lungusa.org/air/envhayfever.html>.

The US National Institute of Allergy and Infectious Diseases (NIAID) has produced an online publication called 'Something in the air: airborne allergens'. It covers a range of allergens, including pollen, dust mite and mould. This is available at:
<http://www.niaid.nih.gov/publications/allergens/title.htm>.

All Allergy is a gateway to a huge range of Web-based information about allergies (although possibly not quite as comprehensive as it claims). It is commercially funded, but editorially independent. The homepage can be found at <http://www.allallergy.net/>.

Headache and migraine

Support group

Migraine Action Association (formerly the British Migraine Association)
178a High Road
Byfleet
West Byfleet
Surrey
KT14 7ED

Tel: 01932 352468
Fax: 01932 351257
E-mail: info@migraine.org.uk
Web page: <http://www.migraine.org.uk/>

Online discussion list
Name of list: **Headache**

Provides a forum for the exchange of information about the various forms of recurring headaches – migraine, cluster, and vascular.

To join this discussion list send the following message:

To: listserv@shsu.edu
Text: subscribe headache *firstname lastname*

Web archive of messages: not available.

Online newsgroup
Name of newsgroup: <news://alt.support.headaches.migraine>

To view the Web archive of messages, go to <http://groups.google.com/> and enter the following: alt.support.headaches.migraine

Suggested summary documents
The Migraine Trust has a section of its Web site devoted to information for migraine sufferers. It includes 'Facts about migraine' and advice on 'Avoiding attacks', available at: <http://www.migrainetrust.org/suffer.htm>.

The American Council for Headache Education has produced a detailed information page called 'Headache facts: what everyone should know'. As well as discussing causes and treatments of a range of different headache types, it also suggests when to see a doctor and offers a range of useful questions to ask. It is available at:
<http://www.achenet.org/news/headfact.php>.

Heart diseases

Support group
British Heart Foundation
14 Fitzhardinge Street
London
W1H 6DH

Tel: 0870 600 6566
Fax: 020 7486 5820
E-mail: n/a
Web page: <http://www.bhf.org.uk/>

Online discussion list
Name of list: **Hearttalk-L**

Discussion and support group for heart patients (and their family and friends).

To join this discussion list send the following message:

To: listserv@maelstrom.stjohns.edu
Text: subscribe hearttalk-l *firstname lastname*

Web archive of messages available at:
<http://maelstrom.stjohns.edu/archives/hearttalk-l.html>

Online newsgroup
Name of newsgroup: <news://sci.med.cardiology>

To view the Web archive of messages, go to <http://groups.google.com/> and enter the following: sci.med.cardiology

Suggested summary documents
The American Heart Association has produced an information page, 'What is heart disease?'. It gives examples of some types of heart disease and provides links to other relevant patient information pages. It is available at:
<http://www.americanheart.org/Patient_Information/hhrt-dis.html>.

Loyola University Health System provides a series of documents on the subject of cardiovascular disease. Topics include anatomy of the heart, signs and symptoms of heart attacks, coronary heart disease, strokes, high blood pressure, and rheumatic heart disease. A link to 'other cardiac conditions' provides a brief overview of more unusual conditions. This information can be downloaded from:
<http://www.luhs.org/health/topics/cardiac/index.htm>.

Hepatitis

Support group

British Liver Trust
Central House
Central Avenue
Ransomes Europark
Ipswich
Suffolk
IP3 9QG

Tel: 0808 800 1000
Fax: 01473 276327
E-mail: info@britishlivertrust.org.uk
Web page: <http://www.britishlivertrust.org.uk/>

Online discussion list

Name of list: **HEPV-L**

This list is primarily intended for people who have been diagnosed with hepatitis of all forms, but is also open to doctors, nurses, or family members.

To join this discussion list send the following message:

To: listserv@sjuvm.stjohns.edu
Text: sub hepv-l *firstname lastname*

Web archive of messages: not available.

Yahoo! Groups include over 40 lists about hepatitis. For more information, go to: <http://dir.groups.yahoo.com/dir/1600061698>.

Online newsgroup

Name of newsgroup: <news://sci.med.diseases.hepatitis>

To view the Web archive of messages, go to <http://groups.google.com/> and enter the following: sci.med.diseases.hepatitis

Suggested summary documents

The British Liver Trust provides online patient information leaflets on a range of subjects, including hepatitis A, hepatitis B and hepatitis C. These can be accessed from the Web site at: <http://www.britishlivertrust.org.uk/publications/index.html>.

The Haemophilia Society offers a detailed guide called 'Hepatitis C: the facts', that covers transmission, tests and treatment, and also includes a section on occupational and employment rights. It can be found on their Web site at: <http://www.haemophilia.org.uk/hepmenu.html>.

Hypertension (high blood pressure)

Support group
British Hypertension Society
Blood Pressure Unit
St George's Hospital Medical School
Cranmer Terrace
London
SW17 0RE

Tel: 020 8725 3412
Fax: 020 8725 2959
E-mail: bhsis@sghms.ac.uk
Web page: <http://www.hyp.ac.uk/bhsinfo/>

See also:
High Blood Pressure Foundation: <http://www.hbpf.org.uk/>

Online discussion list
Name of list: **bloodpressureline**

Provides support and information for patients who have hypertension, or are interested in the effects and treatment of high blood pressure.

To join this discussion list send the following message:

To: bloodpressureline-subscribe@yahoogroups.com
Text: leave blank

Web archive of messages: for members only.

More information available at: <http://groups.yahoo.com/group/bloodpressureline>

Online newsgroup
Though there is no newsgroup devoted exclusively to hypertension, this subject is frequently discussed in both <news://sci.med.cardiology> and <news://alt.support.diet>.

To view the Web archive of messages, go to <http://groups.google.com/> and enter either: sci.med.cardiology *or* alt.support.diet

Suggested summary documents

The British Hypertension Society provides a range of informative leaflets on its Web site. For a general overview, 'Understanding high blood pressure' is highly recommended <http://www.hyp.ac.uk/bhsinfo/understanding.htm>.

The US National Heart, Lung, and Blood Institute has produced a 'High blood pressure' Web site <http://www.nhlbi.nih.gov/hbp/consumer/consumer.html>, which includes information about keeping high blood pressure under control. The American Heart Association also provides patient information – see: <http://www.americanheart.org/hbp/index.jsp>.

Hyperactivity

See **Attention deficit disorder with hyperactivity (ADDH/ADHD).**

Impotence

Support group

Impotence Association
PO Box 10296
London
SW17 9ZH

Tel (Helpline): 020 8767 7791
Fax: 020 8516 7725
E-mail: theia@btinternet.com
Web page: <http://www.impotence.org.uk/>

Online discussion lists

Name of list: **Impotence Support**

A support group for men who suffer from poor or short-lived penile erections, or total impotence.

To join this discussion list send the following message:

To: impotence_support-subscribe@yahoogroups.com
Text: leave blank

Web archive of messages available at:
<http://groups.yahoo.com/group/Impotence_Support>

Name of list: **supportEDpartners**

A moderated discussion group for the partners of men experiencing erectile dysfunction. Due to the sensitive nature of the topic, membership is by approval of the moderators with the intent of maintaining privacy and limiting off topic discussion.

To join this discussion list send the following message:

To: supportedpartners-subscribe@yahoogroups.com
Text: leave blank

Web archive of messages available at:
<http://groups.yahoo.com/group/supportedpartners>

It is necessary to register with Yahoo! Groups <http://groups.yahoo.com/>, but registration is free.

Online newsgroup

Name of newsgroup: <news://alt.support.impotence>

To view the Web archive of messages, go to <http://groups.google.com/> and enter the following: alt.support.impotence

Information about the group in the form of 'Frequently Asked Questions' (and answers) can be found at: <http://www.alt-support-impotence.org/faq.htm>.

Suggested summary documents

The US National Kidney and Urologic Diseases Information Clearinghouse has produced an informative online factsheet, looking at causes of erectile dysfunction, diagnosis and treatment. It can be found at: <http://www.niddk.nih.gov/health/urolog/pubs/impotnce/impotnce.htm>.

Incontinence

Support group

Continence Foundation (Incontinence Information Helpline)
307 Hatton Square
16 Baldwins Gardens
London EC1N 7RJ

Tel: 020 7831 9831
Fax: 020 7404 6876
E-mail: continence-help@dial.pipex.com
Web page: <http://www.continence-foundation.org.uk>

Online discussion lists
Name of list: **INCONT-L**

This list discusses incontinence in all ages, but much discussion centres on 'elder incontinence'.

To join this discussion list send the following message:

To: incont-l-request@maine.maine.edu
Text: subscribe incont-l *firstname lastname*

Web archive of messages: not available.

Name of list: **Incontinence**

This list was established to provide a forum and information exchange for both professionals and patients concerning problems of urinary and facal incontinence. It is a combination of two earlier lists: 'IncontiPro' and 'IncontiList', previously hosted by <http://www.incontinent.com> for professionals and patients respectively.

To join this discussion list send the following message:

To: incontinence-subscribe@yahoogroups.com
Text: leave blank

Web archive of messages and further information available at:
<http://groups.yahoo.com/group/incontinence>

It is necessary to register with Yahoo! Groups <http://groups.yahoo.com/>, but registration is free.

Online newsgroup
Name of newsgroup: <news://alt.support.incontinence>

To view the Web archive of messages, go to <http://groups.google.com/> and enter the following: alt.support.incontinence

Suggested summary documents
The Continence Foundation is developing a very informative Web site which includes information about symptoms and treatments of bladder and bowel problems aimed at the general public: <http://www.continence-foundation.org.uk/docs/framebb.htm>.

Incontact, a UK organisation for people affected by bowel and bladder problems, and their carers, also has a useful site at: <http://www.incontact.demon.co.uk/>. As well as information on bladder and bowel problems, it includes a section on 'news and views', and links to sites about commercial products.

The Simon Foundation for Continence in the US has produced a guide called 'Talking to Your Doctor About Incontinence', available at: <http://www.simonfoundation.org/html/e/reprints/toc.htm>. It includes advice on how to describe your symptoms, what information to bring to the consultation, and how to recognise an 'unacceptable' or 'apathetic' response.

Infertility

Support group

CHILD – The National Infertility Support Network
Charter House
43 St Leonards Road
Bexhill on Sea
East Sussex
TN40 1JA

Tel: 01424 732361
Fax: 01424 731858
E-mail: office@child.org.uk
Web page: <http://www.child.org.uk/>

Online discussion list

Name of list: **ILIST**

Infertility mailing list.

To join this discussion list send the following message:

To: majordomo@acpub.duke.edu
Text: subscribe ilist

Web archive of messages: not available.

For more information, send the message **info ilist to** the same address, or contact the listowner at: owner-ilist@plusnet.org

An extensive list of discussion lists about aspects of infertility can be found at: <http://www.fertilityplus.org/faq/maillists.html>.

Online newsgroups

Name of newsgroup: <news://misc.health.infertility> (for medical discussions only)

Name of newsgroup: <news://alt.infertility> (for all aspects of infertility, including emotional issues)

To view the Web archive of messages, go to <http://groups.google.com/> and enter either: misc.health.infertility *or* alt.infertility

Suggested summary documents

Clear and detailed infertility information pages are available on the Women's Health Information site at <http://www.womens-health.co.uk/infertility.htm>. The pages are maintained by Dr Danny Tucker, a Specialist Registrar in Obstetrics and Gynaecology and a Member of the UK Royal College of Obstetrics & Gynaecology (MRCOG).

The Human Fertilisation and Embryology Association provides patient information about techniques for assisted conception, which includes a section on choosing a clinic. (In the UK, these treatments can be provided only by clinics licensed by the HFEA.) The patient information pages can be found at <http://www.hfea.gov.uk/frame2.htm>.

Irritable bowel syndrome

Support group

IBS Network
Northern General Hospital
Sheffield
S5 7AU

Tel: 0114 2611531
Fax: n/a
E-mail: penny@ibsnetwork.org.uk
Web page: <http://www.ibsnetwork.org.uk/>

Online discussion list

Yahoo! Groups <http://groups.yahoo.com/> hosts several discussion groups about IBS. It is necessary to register with the service, but registration is free. The list with most subscribers is:

Name of list: **IBS_News**

'The complete resource for the IBS sufferer!'

To join this discussion list send the following message:

To: ibs_news-subscribe@yahoogroups.com
Text: leave blank

Web archive of messages available at:
<http://groups.yahoo.com/group/IBS_News>

Online newsgroup

Name of newsgroup: <news://alt.support.ibs>

To view the Web archive of messages, go to <http://groups.google.com/> and enter the following: alt.support.ibs

Suggested summary documents

The Digestive Disorders Foundation provides a range of clear and helpful online patient information leaflets, including one for IBS: <http://www.digestivedisorders.org.uk/leaflets/ibs.html>.

The US National Digestive Diseases Information Clearinghouse (NDDIC) provides an overview in the form of questions and answers about causes, symptoms, diagnosis and treatment. It is available at: <http://www.niddk.nih.gov/health/digest/pubs/irrbowel/irrbowel.htm>.

Kidney diseases

Support group

National Kidney Federation
6 Stanley Street
Worksop
England
S81 7HX

Tel (Helpline): 0845 6010209
Tel: 01909 487795
Fax: 01909 481723
E-mail: mks@kidney.org.uk
Web page: <http://www.kidney.org.uk/>

Online discussion list

Name of list: **KIDNEY-ONC**

An unmoderated list, sponsored by the US National Kidney Cancer Association. It is intended for patients, family, friends, researchers and physicians, to discuss clinical and non-clinical issues and advances pertaining to kidney cancer.

To join this discussion list send the following message:

To: listserv@medinfo.org

Text: subscribe kidney-onc *firstname lastname*

Web archive of messages available at: <http://listserv.acor.org/archives/kidney-onc.html>

Online newsgroup

Name of newsgroup: <news://alt.support.kidney-disease>

To view the Web archive of messages, go to <http://groups.google.com/> and enter the following: alt.support.kidney-disease

Suggested summary documents

The Kidney Patient Guide is a very useful Web site providing information for renal patients, their partners and families, healthcare professionals and anyone else who is interested in kidney disease. As well as information on physical aspects of kidney failure, it also addresses wider issues such as emotional, social and financial implications. This site can be found at: <http://www.kidneypatientguide.org.uk/>.

The Royal Infirmary of Edinburgh Renal Unit has produced EdRenINFO, a source of information about kidney diseases for patients, or for doctors who are not renal specialists. Information is provided at two levels: 'Get info', which is quite basic; and 'Get more info', which is more detailed. These resources are available at: <http://renux.dmed.ed.ac.uk/EdREN/EdRenINFOhome.html>.

The US National Institute of Diabetes and Digestive and Kidney Disorders (NIDDK) <http://www.niddk.nih.gov/health/kidney/kidney.htm> also provides a range of online publications, covering kidney function as well as various medical conditions.

Leukaemia

See also **Cancer.**

Support group

Leukaemia Research Fund
43 Great Ormond Street
London
WC1N 3JJ

Tel: 020 7405 0101
Fax: 020 7242 1488
E-mail: info@lrf.org.uk
Web page: <http://dspace.dial.pipex.com/lrf-//index.htm>

Online discussion lists

The American Association of Cancer Online Resources (ACOR) hosts several mailing lists about leukaemia, for example:

Name of list: **ALL-L (Acute Lymphocytic Leukemia – general list)**

An unmoderated discussion list for patients and others for discussion of clinical and non-clinical issues and advances pertaining to acute lymphocytic leukaemia in adults.

To join this discussion list send the following message:

To: listserv@listserv.acor.org
Text: subscribe all-l

Web archive of messages available at: <http://listserv.acor.org/archives/all-l.html>

The other ACOR leukaemia lists are: **AML** (acute myelogenous leukemia); **CLL** (chronic lymphocytic leukemia); **CML** (chronic myelogenous leukemia); **HAIRY-CELL** (hairy cell leukemia list); **ALL-KIDS** (childhood acute lymphoblastic leukemia); **PED-ALL** (pediatric acute lymphocytic leukemia). For more information, send the following message:

To: listserv@listserv.acor.org
Text: info *listname*

Online newsgroup

Name of newsgroup: <news://alt.support.cancer>

To view the Web archive of messages, go to <http://groups.google.com/> and enter the following: alt.support.cancer

Suggested summary documents

As part of a range of online booklets, the charity CancerBACUP provides information on four types of leukaemia: acute lymphoblastic leukaemia; acute myeloblastic leukaemia; chronic lymphocytic leukaemia; and chronic myeloid leukaemia. They are available at <http://www.cancerbacup.org.uk/info/specific-cancers.htm>.

As part of its CancerNet service, the US National Cancer Institute provides very detailed information on various types of leukaemia. It includes a section on 'Coping', which looks at complications of cancer and side effects of treatment. It can be found at:
<http://cancernet.nci.nih.gov/Cancer_Types/Leukemia.shtml>. This site also includes a useful overview of leukaemia, available at:
<http://cancernet.nci.nih.gov/wyntk_pubs/leukemia.htm>.

Lung cancer

See also **Cancer.**

Support group
Roy Castle Lung Cancer Foundation
200 London Road
Liverpool
L3 9TA

Tel: 0151 794 8800
Fax: 0151 794 8888
E-mail: foundation@roycastle.org
Web page: <http://www.roycastle.org/>

Online discussion list
Name of list: **LUNG-ONC: The Lung Cancer Online Support Group**

LUNG-ONC is an unmoderated discussion list for patients and others to discuss clinical and non-clinical issues and advances pertaining to lung cancers.

To join this discussion list send the following message:

To: listserv@listserv.acor.org
Text: subscribe lung-onc

Web archive of messages available at: <http://listserv.acor.org/archives/lung-onc.html>

For more information, send the following message:

To: listserv@listserv.acor.org
Text: info lung-onc

Online newsgroup

Name of newsgroup: <news://alt.support.cancer>

To view the Web archive of messages, go to <http://groups.google.com/> and enter the following: alt.support.cancer

Suggested summary documents

Lung Cancer Online <http://www.lungcanceronline.org/> is an extremely informative gateway to lung cancer resources created for the benefit of people with lung cancer and their families. The editor, Karen Parles, is a 'mother, wife and librarian who was diagnosed with lung cancer in January 1998'.

The Royal Marsden Hospital is developing an excellent 'Patient Information Series', providing information about different types of cancer, treatments, living with the side effects and adjusting to the changes caused by cancer. The content of the booklets and leaflets is based on common questions asked by patients and all titles are regularly reviewed and updated. The booklet for lung cancer can be found at: <http://www.royalmarsden.org/patientinfo/booklets/lung_cancer/index.asp>.

As part of a range of online booklets, the charity CancerBACUP provides comprehensive information on 'Understanding cancer of the lung', covering causes, symptoms, diagnosis, types of treatment and further reading <http://www.cancerbacup.org.uk/info/lung.htm>. They also provide a fact sheet about an uncommon type of cancer known as mesothelioma: <http://www.cancerbacup.org.uk/info/mesothelioma.htm>.

Lupus

Support group

Lupus UK
St James House
Eastern Road
Romford
RM1 3NH

Tel: 01708 731251
Fax: 01708 731252
E-mail: headoffice@lupus-uk.freeserve.co.uk
Web page: <http://www.geocities.com/HotSprings/2911/>

Online discussion list

Hamline University hosts a Lupus Home Page <http://www.hamline.edu/lupus/> and three lupus mailing lists.

Name of lists: **LUPUS-L, LUPUS-R, LUPUS-S**

LUPUS-L is concerned with the medical concerns of patients, **LUPUS-R** is concerned with research, and **LUPUS-S** is concerned with the social and support needs of lupus patients.

To subscribe to any of these lists, send the following message:

To: listproc@piper.hamline.edu
Text: subscribe *list-name your name*

Web archive of messages and further information can be found at: <http://wwww.hamline.edu/lupus/listproc.html>

Online newsgroup

Name of newsgroup: <news://alt.support.lupus>

To view the Web archive of messages, go to <http://groups.google.com/> and enter the following: alt.support.lupus

Suggested summary documents

The Arthritis Research Campaign has produced a very informative online information leaflet about lupus <http://www.arc.org.uk/about_arth/booklets/6023/6023.htm>. It describes how lupus can affect various parts of the body, looks at diagnosis and treatment, and offers advice on living with the condition.

The Lupus Foundation of America provides a detailed overview in the form of 'Commonly asked questions about lupus' (with answers). This can be found at: <http://www.lupus.org/lupusfaq.html>.

The US National Institute of Arthritis and Musculoskeletal and Skin Diseases (NIAMS) has produced an online booklet on systemic lupus erythematosus, which defines various types of lupus and describes causes, symptoms, diagnosis and treatment. It can be viewed at: <http://www.nih.gov/niams/healthinfo/slehandout/>.

Lyme disease

Support group

British Lyme Disease Foundation
PO Box 110
Tunbridge Wells
Kent
TN1 1WY

Tel: n/a
Fax: n/a
E-mail: spud@wadhurst.demon.co.uk
Web page: <http://www.wadhurst.demon.co.uk/lyme/>

Online discussion list

Yahoo! Groups hosts about 20 discussion lists on Lyme Disease – see:
<http://dir.groups.yahoo.com/dir/Health_Wellness/Support/Illnesses/
Lyme_Disease>.

Details of a UK-based list are given below.

Name of list: **lymearduk**

The list aims to bring together those with knowledge of, experience of, or
difficulties with Lyme and related disorders in order to promote awareness of
tick-borne infectious disease.

To join this discussion list send the following message:

To: lymearduk-subscribe@yahoogroups.com
Text: leave blank

Web archive of messages available at:
<http://groups.yahoo.com/group/lymearduk>

Online newsgroup

Name of newsgroup: <news://sci.med.diseases.lyme>

To view the Web archive of messages, go to <http://groups.google.com/> and
enter the following: sci.med.diseases.lyme

Suggested summary documents

The Lyme Disease Network <http://www.lymenet.org/> is a US-based non-
profit foundation dedicated to the education of the public about the

prevention and treatment of Lyme disease. The Web site contains general information about the diagnosis, symptoms and treatment of Lyme disease, as well as links to news items about the disease.

The Association of Medical Microbiologists provides a brief overview on its Web site at: <http://www.amm.co.uk/pubs/fa_lyme.htm>. More detailed information can be found on the Web site of the US Lyme Disease Foundation at: <http://www.lyme.org/otherdis/ld.html>.

Lymphoma

See also **Cancer.**

Support group
Lymphoma Association (Formerly the Hodgkin's Disease and Lymphoma Association)
PO Box 386
Aylesbury
Bucks
HP20 2GA

Tel: 0808 808 5555
E-mail: n/a
Web page: <http://www.lymphoma.org.uk/>

Online discussion lists
Name of list: **HODGKINS (Hodgkin's Lymphoma Support Group)**

To join this discussion list send the following message:

To: listserv@listserv.acor.org
Text: subscribe hodgkins

Web archive of messages available at:
<http://listserv.acor.org/archives/hodgkins.html>

Name of list: **NHL (Non Hodgkin's Lymphoma Support Group)**

To join this discussion list send the following message:

To: listserv@listserv.acor.org
Text: subscribe nhl

Web archive of messages available at:
<http://listserv.acor.org/archives/nhl.html>

Online newsgroup

There is not a group specifically about lymphoma, but there are two general newsgroups concerned with cancer: <news://alt.support.cancer> and <news://sci.med.diseases.cancer>.

To view the Web archives of messages, go to <http://groups.google.com/> and enter either: alt.support.cancer *or* sci.med.diseases.cancer

Suggested summary documents

The Lymphoma Association provides a useful range of free publications on lymphomas, their treatments and related issues. For details, see <http://www.lymphoma.org.uk/support/index.htm>.

The Lymphoma Information Network <http://lymphomainfo.net/lymphoma.html> is hosted by Mike Barela, who is a Hodgkin's lymphoma survivor. It has two aims: 'to put a bit of humanity and understanding to this disease and to gather lymphoma information and resources in one place'.

Mad cow disease

See **Creutzfeldt–Jakob disease (CJD).**

Manic depression

See **Bipolar disorder (manic depression).**

Melanoma

See also **Cancer.**

Support group

There is not a UK support group specifically for melanoma, but there are several cancer support groups, for example:

CancerBACUP
3 Bath Place
Rivington Street
London
EC2A 3JR

Tel: 0808 800 1234
Fax: 020 7696 9002
E-mail: info@cancerbacup.org
Web page: <http://www.cancerbacup.org.uk/>

Online discussion list
Name of list: **MEL-L**

A support group for patients, care-givers, doctors and researchers.

To join this discussion list send the following message:

To: listserv@maelstrom.stjohns.edu
Text: subscribe mel-l

Web archive of messages available at:
<http://maelstrom.stjohns.edu/archives/mel-l.html>

Online newsgroup
Name of newsgroup: <news://alt.support.cancer>

To view the Web archive of messages, go to <http://groups.google.com/> and enter the following: alt.support.cancer

Suggested summary documents
CancerBACUP provides an informative online booklet called 'Understanding malignant melanoma' which covers causes, symptoms and treatment. It also looks at follow-up treatment and suggests useful organisations and background reading. It can be found at:
<http://www.cancerbacup.org.uk/info/melanoma.htm>.

The US National Cancer Institute provides clear and detailed information in its patient information page 'What you need to know about melanoma' <http://cancernet.nci.nih.gov/wyntk_pubs/melanoma.htm>.

The Melanoma Patients' Information Page (MPIP) is a non-commercial site founded to provide support and information to melanoma patients and their carers. It aims to provide up-to-date high-quality information from reputable sources. The address is: <http://www.mpip.org/>.

Ménière's disease

Support group

Royal National Institute for Deaf People (RNID)
19–23 Featherstone Street
London
EC1Y 8SL

Tel: 0808 808 0123
Fax: 020 7296 8199
E-mail: helpline@rnid.org.uk
Web page: <http://www.rnid.org.uk/>

There is a support group for Ménière's disease, but it does not have a Web site:

The Ménière's Society
98 Maybury Road
Woking
GU21 5HX.

Tel: 01483 740597
Fax: 01483 755441
E-mail: info@menieres-uk.demon.co.uk

Online discussion list

Name of list: **Menieres**

A mailing list for patients, their families, and medical professionals interested in Ménière's disease.

To join this discussion list send the following message:

To: menieres@smtp.cochlea.com
Text: subscribe menieres *firstname lastname*

Web archive of messages available at: <http://www.cochlea.com>

Online newsgroup

There is not a group devoted to Ménière's disease, but the symptoms of tinnitus and hearing loss are discussed in <news://alt.support.tinnitus> and <news://alt.support.hearing-loss>.

To view the Web archives of messages, go to <http://groups.google.com/> and enter either: alt.support.tinnitus *or* alt.support.hearing-loss

Suggested summary documents

The RNID provides a fact sheet on Ménière's disease, concentrating on symptoms and how to manage them <http://www.rnid.org.uk/html/info_factsheets_med_menieres_disease.htm>.

The US National Institute on Deafness and Other Communication Disorders has produced a patient information leaflet called 'Because you asked about Ménière's disease'. It includes links to background information about hearing and balance. It can be viewed at: <http://www.nidcd.nih.gov/health/pubs_hb/meniere.htm>.

Meningitis

See also **Encephalitis.**

Support group

National Meningitis Trust
Fern House
Bath Road
Stroud
Gloucestershire
GL5 3TJ

Tel (24 hr Helpline): 0845 6000 800
Tel: 01453 768000
Fax: 01453 768001
E-mail: support@meningitis-trust.org.uk
Web page: <http://www.meningitis-trust.org.uk/>

Online discussion list

Name of list: **Meningitis Circle (Meni Circle)**

An e-mail based support group for parents of children who were deafened by meningitis. Most of the children use cochlear implants, or are being evaluated for a cochlear implant. Subscription requires the approval of the list owner.

To join this discussion list send the following message:

To: menicircle-subscribe@topica.com
Text: not specified

Web archive of messages: available to subscribers only.

Online newsgroup

There is no newsgroup specifically about meningitis, but it has been discussed in a more general list about children's health.

Name of newsgroup: <news://misc.kids.health>

To view the Web archive of messages, go to <http://groups.google.com.> and enter the following: misc.kids.health

Suggested summary documents

The Meningitis Research Foundation hosts an informative Web site at <http://www.meningitis.org.uk>. Click on 'About Meningitis' to obtain a brief overview, including information about symptoms of meningitis and septicaemia, vaccination, and a description of the 'tumbler test' for septicaemia. Similarly, the National Meningitis Trust provides a range of information on its Web site at <http://www.meningitis-trust.org.uk/>. The link to 'What is Meningitis' leads to information about different types of meningitis, including symptoms, treatment and prevention.

Migraine

See **Headache and migraine.**

Miscarriage

See under **Bereavement**; also Chapter 10.

Mouth, cancer of

See **Oral cancer.**

Multiple sclerosis

Support group

Multiple Sclerosis Society
25 Effie Road
London
SW6 1EE

Tel (Helpline): 0808 800 8000
Tel: 020 7610 7171
Fax: 020 7736 9861

E-mail: info@mssociety.org.uk
Web page: <http://www.mssociety.org.uk/>

Online discussion list
Name of list: **MSLIST-L**

Multiple Sclerosis discussion list.

To join this discussion list send the following message:

To: listserv@techunix.technion.ac.il
Text: subscribe mslist-l

Web archive of messages available at:
<http://techunix.technion.ac.il/archives/mslist-l.html>

Online newsgroup
Name of newsgroup: <news://uk.people.support.mult-sclerosis>

To view the Web archives of messages, go to <http://groups.google.com/>
and enter the following: uk.people.support.mult-sclerosis

Suggested summary documents
The Multiple Sclerosis Society has published a collection of useful documents
on its Web site, a list of which can be found at:
<http://www.mssociety.org.uk/publications/pubslist.htm>.

The US National Institute of Neurological Disorders and Stroke provides an
online brochure called 'Multiple sclerosis: hope through research'. It covers
causes, symptoms, diagnosis and possible therapies. It can be found at:
<http://www.ninds.nih.gov/health_and_medical/pubs/multiple_sclerosis.htm>.

Jooly's Joint is a free global support network (10,000 members) for people
with MS, run by British women with MS. For more information point your
browser at: <http://www.mswebpals.org/>.

Muscular dystrophy

Support group
Muscular Dystrophy Group
7–11 Prescott Place
London
SW4 6BS

Tel: 020 7720 8055
Fax: 020 7498 0670
E-mail: info@muscular-dystrophy.org
Web page: <http://www.muscular-dystrophy.org/>

Online discussion list
Name of list: **MD-List**

A mailing list for information about muscular dystrophy and related neuro-muscular diseases, intended for patients, family, and friends.

To join this discussion list send the following message:

To: md-list-request@basix.com
Text: subscribe

Web archive of messages available at: <http://www.mdrespite.org/md-list/>

The list owner can be contacted by e-mail at: rich@mdrespite.org

Online newsgroup
Name of newsgroup: <news://alt.support.musc-dystrophy>

To view the Web archives of messages, go to <http://groups.google.com/> and enter the following: alt.support.musc-dystrophy

Suggested summary documents
The Muscular Dystrophy Group has produced a range of useful fact sheets. They can be viewed in PDF format (which require an Adobe Acrobat Reader – see Chapter 3) or in text format. A list of fact sheets about specific conditions can be found at: <http://www.muscular-dystrophy.org/information/Key%20facts/advice.html>.

The Muscular Dystrophy Association in the US also provides a range of freely available Web publications. 'Facts about muscular dystrophy' provides a useful overview, and includes a list of 'major characteristics of the 9 muscular dystrophies'. It is available at: <http://www.mdausa.org/publications/fa-md-9.html>.

Myalgic encephalomyelitis (ME)

See **Chronic Fatigue Syndrome (CFS).**

Obsessive compulsive disorder

Support group
Obsessive Action
Aberdeen Centre
22–24 Highbury Grove
London
N5 2EA

Tel: 020 7226 4000
Fax: 020 7288 0828
E-mail: obsessive-action@demon.co.uk
Web page: <http://www.obsessive-action.demon.co.uk/>

Online discussion list
Name of list: **OCD-L**

The aim of this list is to support discussion of obsessive-compulsive disorders.

To join this discussion list send the following message:

To: listserv@vm.marist.edu
Text: subscribe ocd-l *firstname lastname*

Web archive of messages: not available.

Online newsgroup
Name of newsgroup: <news://alt.support.ocd>

To view the Web archive of messages, go to <http://groups.google.com/> and enter the following: alt.support.ocd

Suggested summary documents
The mental health charity Mind has produced a booklet called 'Understanding obsessive compulsive disorder'. This is available at: <http://www.mind.org.uk/information/understanding/ocd/understanding_obsessive_compulsive_disorder.asp>.

'Again and again', a collection of obsessive compulsive disorder Web sites, can be found at: <http://www.interlog.com/~calex/ocd/index.html>.

Oral cancer

See also **Cancer.**

Support group

There is no UK support group specifically for oral cancer, but there are several organisations concerned with cancer generally. For example:

CancerBACUP
3 Bath Place
Rivington Street
London
EC2A 3JR

Tel: 0808 800 1234
Fax: 020 7696 9002
E-mail: info@cancerbacup.org
Web page: <http://www.cancerbacup.org.uk/>

Online discussion list

Name of list: **ORAL-ONC**

ORAL-ONC is an unmoderated discussion list for patients, family, friends, researchers and physicians, to discuss clinical and non-clinical issues and advances relating to oral cancers.

To join this discussion list send the following message:

To: listserv@listserv.acor.org
Text: subscribe oral-onc

Web archive of messages available at: <http://listserv.acor.org/archives/oral-onc.html>

Online newsgroup

Name of newsgroup: <news://alt.support.cancer>

To view the Web archive of messages, go to <http://groups.google.com/> and enter the following: alt.support.cancer

Suggested summary documents

As part of their booklet series, CancerBACUP has produced 'Understanding cancer of the mouth and throat'. As well as a clear explanation of symptoms, diagnosis and treatment, it provides links to information about other useful organisations. The booklet can be found at: <http://www.cancerbacup.org.uk/info/mouth.htm>.

Clear and detailed information is available from CancerNet, a service provided by the US National Cancer Institute. 'What you need to know about oral cancer' is available at: <http://cancernet.nci.nih.gov/wyntk_pubs/oral.htm>.

The American Cancer Society provides an online 'Cancer Resource Center' <http://www3.cancer.org/cancerinfo/>. Specific types of cancer can be selected from a drop-down list. Information is provided about the nature of cancer, its causes, and risk factors, as well as strategies for prevention and early detection, diagnostic techniques and treatment options.

Osteoporosis

Support group
National Osteoporosis Society
PO Box 10
Radstock
Bath
BA3 3YB

Tel: 01761 472 721
Fax: 01761 471104
E-mail: info@nos.org.uk
Web page: <http://www.nos.org.uk/>

Online discussion list
Name of list: **OSTEO-P**

OSTEO-P is an unmoderated discussion list for patients, family, friends, researchers, and physicians, to discuss clinical and non-clinical issues and advances relating to osteoporosis.

To join this discussion list send the following message:

To: listserv@listserv.acor.org
Text: subscribe osteo-p

Web archive of messages available at: <http://listserv.acor.org/archives/osteo-p.html>.

Online newsgroup

Name of newsgroup: <news://sci.med.diseases.osteoporosis>

To view the Web archive of messages, go to <http://groups.google.com/> and enter the following: sci.med.diseases.osteoporosis

Suggested summary documents

The National Osteoporosis Society provides a useful overview on its Web site at <http://www.nos.org.uk/gener.htm>. Other pages cover prevention, including dietary advice, and treatment.

An informative American site can be found at <http://www.osteo.org/>. This is the National Institutes of Health Osteoporosis and Related Bone Diseases – National Resource Center. It includes a range of 'bone health information', and also provides 'research bibliographies' compiled from MEDLINE (see Chapter 5) and 'bone links' to other useful sites.

Ovarian cancer

See also **Cancer.**

Support group

Ovacome
St Bartholomew's Hospital
West Smithfield
London
EC1A 7BE

Tel: 07071 781861 (NB mobile rates apply, but they will call back.)
Fax: n/a
E-mail: ovacome@ovacome.org.uk
Web page: <http://www.ovacome.org.uk/ovacome/>

Online discussion list

Name of list: **OVARIAN**

This list provides various kinds of support relating to ovarian cancer and related conditions, including ovarian cysts. Reproductive issues are not covered except as they relate to ovarian cancer. For more information, contact the list managers by e-mail at:
Ovarian-request@listserv.acor.org

To join this discussion list send the following message:

To: listserv@listserv.acor.org
Text: subscribe ovarian

Web archive of messages available at: <http://listserv.acor.org/archives/ovarian.html>

Online newsgroup

Name of newsgroup: <news://alt.support.cancer>

To view the Web archive of messages, go to <http://groups.google.com/> and enter the following: alt.support.cancer

Suggested summary documents

As part of their booklet series, CancerBACUP have produced 'Understanding cancer of the ovary'. As well as a clear explanation of symptoms, diagnosis and treatment, it provides links to information about other useful organisations. The booklet can be found at:
<http://www.cancerbacup.org.uk/info/ovary.htm>.

Clear and detailed information is available from CancerNet, a service provided by the US National Cancer Institute. 'What you need to know about ovarian cancer' is available at: <http://cancernet.nci.nih.gov/wyntk_pubs/ovarian.htm >.

The American Cancer Society provides an online 'Cancer Resource Center': <http://www3.cancer.org/cancerinfo/>. Specific types of cancer can be selected from a drop-down list. Information is provided about the nature of cancer, its causes and risk factors, as well as strategies for prevention and early detection, diagnostic techniques and treatment options.

Pancreatic cancer

See also **Cancer.**

Support group

There is not a UK support group specifically for pancreatic cancer, but there are several cancer support groups, for example:

CancerBACUP
3 Bath Place
Rivington Street
London
EC2A 3JR

Tel: 0808 800 1234
Fax: 020 7696 9002
E-mail: info@cancerbacup.org
Web page: <http://www.cancerbacup.org.uk/>

Online discussion list
Name of list: **PANCREAS-ONC**

An unmoderated discussion list for patients, friends, researchers and physicians, to discuss clinical and non-clinical issues and advances relating to pancreatic cancer.

To join this discussion list send the following message:

To: listserv@listserv.acor.org
Text: subscribe pancreas-onc

Web archive of messages available at: <http://listserv.acor.org/archives/pancreas-onc.html>

Online newsgroup
Name of newsgroup: <news://alt.support.cancer>

To view the Web archive of messages, go to <http://groups.google.com/> and enter the following: alt.support.cancer

Suggested summary documents
As part of its excellent booklet series, the charity Cancer BACUP has produced 'Understanding cancer of the pancreas'. As well as explaining causes, symptoms, diagnosis and treatment, it discusses the emotional shock of a cancer diagnosis, and provides information about useful organisations and 'recommended reading'. It can be found at:
<http://www.cancerbacup.org.uk/info/pancreas.htm>.

The Digestive Disorders Foundation provides a brief overview in its leaflet 'Cancer of the pancreas':
<http://www.digestivedisorders.org.uk/leaflets/pancreaz.html>.

As part of its CancerNet service, the US National Cancer Institute provides detailed information on cancer of the pancreas, including symptoms, treatment and follow-up care. It includes links to related online booklets, and a dictionary of specialised terms. It can be found at:
<http://cancernet.nci.nih.gov/wyntk_pubs/pancreas.htm>.

Parkinson's disease

Support group

Parkinson's Disease Society
215 Vauxhall Bridge Road
London
SW1V 1EJ

Tel: 020 7931 8080
Fax: 020 7233 9908
E-mail: enquiries@parkinsons.org.uk
Web page: <http://www.parkinsons.org.uk/>

Online discussion lists

Name of list: **PARKINSN**

This is described as 'the main worldwide mailing list about Parkinson's disease'. It has over 1500 members and the list generates around 20 to 30 messages a day.

To join this discussion list send the following message:

To: listserv@listserv.utoronto.ca
Text: sub parkinsn *firstname lastname*

Web archive of messages available at:
<http://james.parkinsons.org.uk/PARKINSN/search.htm>

Further information can be found at:
<http://james.parkinsons.org.uk/Lists/parkinsn.htm>

A list devoted to UK users is **PDUK**. Further information can be found at: <http://www.coles.org.uk/Current_Projects/Lists/pduk.htm>.

Online newsgroup

Name of newsgroup: <news://alt.support.disorders.neurological>

To view the Web archive of messages, go to <http://groups.google.com/> and enter the following: alt.support.disorders.neurological

Suggested summary documents

The US National Institute of Neurological Disorders and Stroke has produced a brief overview of Parkinson's, which can be found at: <http://www.ninds.nih.gov/health_and_medical/disorders/parkinsons_disease.htm>. More detailed information can be found at a related page 'Parkinson's disease — hope through research' <http://www.ninds.nih.gov/health_and_medical/pubs/parkinson_disease_htr.htm>. As well as looking at symptoms, diagnosis and treatment, it describes current research.

The Adrienne Coles Memorial Trust (ACMT) is a private trust dedicated to Parkinson's disease information on the Internet. For more information see <http://www.coles.org.uk/>.

Post-traumatic stress disorder (PTSD)

Support group

Trauma Aftercare Trust (TACT)
Buttfields
1 The Farthings
Withington
Gloucestershire
GL54 4DF

Tel (Helpline): 0800 1696814
Tel: 01242 890306
Fax: 01242 890498
E-mail: tact@tacthq.demon.co.uk
Web page: <http://www.tacthq.demon.co.uk/>

Online discussion list

Name of list: **PTSD**

PTSD is a support and discussion list for 'ALL people with disabilities (pwd) who have or think they may have post-traumatic stress disorder (PTSD)' – as well as family, friends and professionals.

To join this discussion list send the following message:

To: listserv@maelstrom.stjohns.edu
Text: subscribe ptsd

Web archive of messages available at:
<http://maelstrom.stjohns.edu/archives/ptsd.html>

Online newsgroup

Name of newsgroup: <news://alt.support.trauma-ptsd>

To view the Web archive of messages, go to <http://groups.google.com/> and enter the following: alt.support.trauma-ptsd

Suggested summary documents

The Northumberland Mental Health Trust (Department of Psychological Therapies and Research) has produced a range of self-help guides that are available on their Web site in PDF format (see Chapter 3). The booklet on post-traumatic stress describes typical reactions to traumatic incidents and offers practical suggestions for coping <http://www.northumberland-haz.org.uk/selfhelp/default.htm>.

The American National Center for PTSD hosts a page called 'Facts about PTSD' <http://www.ncptsd.org/facts/index.html>, which provides a wide range of fact sheets aimed at different audiences.

Internet Mental Health is an award-winning free encyclopaedia of mental health information, designed by Canadian psychiatrist Dr Phillip Long. It provides information about a range of disorders, treatment and research information, as well as links to other sites. Go to the page <http://www.mentalhealth.com/fr20.html> and select 'post-traumatic stress disorder' from the list.

Prostate cancer

See also **Cancer.**

Support group

Prostate Cancer Charity
3, Angel Walk
Hammersmith
London
W6 9HX

Tel: 0845 300 8383
Fax: 020 8222 7639
E-mail: info@prostate-cancer.org.uk
Web page: <http://www.prostate-cancer.org.uk/>

Online discussion list

Name of list: **PROSTATE (Prostate Problems Mailing List)**

This list is managed by volunteers and hosted by ACOR, the Association of Cancer On-Line Resources, a private foundation that receives no government funding. The objective of the PPML is 'to provide a forum for the newly diagnosed and "been there" prostate cancer (PCa)(CaP) survivors, together with loved ones and helpful professionals, to discuss and exchange information concerning PCa'.

To join this discussion list send the following message:

To: listserv@listserv.acor.org
Text: subscribe prostate

Web archive of messages available at:
<http://listserv.acor.org/archives/prostate.html>

Online newsgroups
Name of newsgroup: <news://alt.support.cancer.prostate>
Name of newsgroup: <news://sci.med.prostate.cancer>

To view the Web archives of messages, go to <http://groups.google.com/>
and enter either: alt.support.cancer.prostate *or* group:sci.med.prostate.cancer

Suggested summary documents
As part of its excellent booklet series, the charity Cancer BACUP has produced
'Understanding cancer of the prostate'. As well as explaining causes,
symptoms, diagnosis and treatment, it discusses the emotional shock of a
cancer diagnosis, and provides information about useful organisations and
'recommended reading'. It can be found at:
<http://www.cancerbacup.org.uk/info/prostate.htm>.

As part of its CancerNet service, the US National Cancer Institute provides
detailed information on prostate cancer, including symptoms, treatment and
follow-up care. It includes links to related online booklets, and a dictionary of
specialised terms. This information is available at:
<http://cancernet.nci.nih.gov/wyntk_pubs/prostate.htm>.

Information for men who are thinking about having a screening test for
prostate cancer, called the PSA test, can be found at:
<http://www.york.ac.uk/inst/crd/em22b.htm>.

Psoriasis

Support groups
The Psoriasis Association
Milton House
7 Milton Street
Northampton
NN2 7JG

Tel: 01604 711129
Fax: 01604 792894
E-mail: n/a
Web address: <http://www.timewarp.demon.co.uk/psoriasis.html>

Psoriatic Arthropathy Alliance
PO Box 111
St Albans
AL2 3JQ

Tel: 01923 672837
Fax: 01923 672837
E-mail: info@paalliance.org
Web page: <http://www.paalliance.org/>

Online discussion list

Yahoo! Groups hosts nearly 40 different lists concerned with psoriasis – see <http://groups.yahoo.com/search?query=psoriasis>. Details for a general list are provided.

Name of list: **psoriasis_support**

To join this discussion list send the following message:

To: psoriasis_support-subscribe@yahoogroups.com
Text: leave blank

Web archive of messages: for members only.

For more information, see: <http://groups.yahoo.com/group/ psoriasis_support>

Online newsgroup

Name of newsgroup: <news://alt.support.skin-diseases.psoriasis>

To view the Web archive of messages, go to <http://groups.google.com/> and enter the following: alt.support.skin-diseases.psoriasis

Suggested summary documents

The British Association of Dermatologists provides a range of patient information leaflets about skin disorders. A description of psoriasis and information about treatment can be found at: <http://www.bad.org.uk/ staticpages/1/patient/psoriasis.html>.

More detailed information about different types of psoriasis can be found at <http://www.psoriasis.org/b200.htm>, provided by the US National Psoriasis Foundation.

Sarcoidosis

Support group

Though there is no UK support group specifically for sarcoidosis, the British Lung Foundation is able to provide advice and support.

British Lung Foundation
78 Hatton Garden
London
EC1N 8LD

Tel: 020 7831 5831
Fax: 020 7831 5832
E-mail: blf@britishlungfoundation.com
Web page: <http://www.lunguk.org/>

Online discussion list

Name of list: **Sarcoidnet** – The London Ontario Sarcoidosis Information Connection

This Canadian-based Web site <http://www.geocities.com/HotSprings/Villa/6542/> hosts this sarcoidosis discussion list. Join this forum by entering your e-mail address where prompted.

Online newsgroup

At the time of writing, there was not a group devoted to sarcoidosis, but it has been discussed in a variety of groups, particularly <news://sci.med.diseases.lyme>.

To view the Web archive of messages, go to <http://groups.google.com/> and enter the following: sci.med.diseases.lyme

Suggested summary documents

The US National Heart, Lung, and Blood Institute provides a detailed overview, including illustrations and a glossary. It can be found at:<http://www.nhlbi.nih.gov/health/public/lung/other/sarcoidosis/index.htm>.

The British Association of Dermatologists provides a brief but clear description. Go to <http://www.skinhealth.co.uk/index.cfm>, then click on 'Patient Information', and then on 'Sarcoidosis'.

Schizophrenia

Support groups

National Schizophrenia Fellowship
30 Tabernacle Street
London
EC2A 4DD

Tel: 020 8974 6814
Fax: 020 7330 9102
E-mail: info@nsf.org.uk
Web page: <http://www.nsf.org.uk/>

Schizophrenia Association of Great Britain
'Bryn Hyfryd'
The Crescent
Bangor
Gwynedd
LL57 2AG

Tel & fax: 01248.354048
E-mail: sagb@btinternet.com
Web page: <http://www.btinternet.com/~sagb/>

Online discussion list

Name of list: **SCHIZOPH**

To join this discussion list send the following message:

To: listserv@maelstrom.stjohns.edu
Text: subscribe schizoph

Web archive of messages available at:
<http://maelstrom.stjohns.edu/archives/schizoph.html>

Online newsgroup

Name of newsgroup: <news://alt.support.schizophrenia>

To view the Web archive of messages, go to <http://groups.google.com/> and enter the following: alt.support.schizophrenia

Suggested summary documents

The Royal College of Psychiatrists has produced an excellent series of leaflets

for the general public on common mental health issues. The leaflet about schizophrenia can be found at:
<http://www.rcpsych.ac.uk/public/help/schiz/sch_frame.htm>.

The Mental Health Foundation has also produced a range of very informative booklets. 'Understanding schizophrenia' is available at: <http://www. mentalhealth.org.uk/bkuschizoph.htm>. The mental health charity Mind has also produced a booklet called 'Understanding schizophrenia' <http://www.mind.org.uk/information/understanding/schizophrenia/ understanding_schizophrenia.asp>.

Scleroderma

Support group
Raynaud's & Scleroderma Association
112 Crewe Road
Alsager
Cheshire
ST7 2JA

Tel: 01270 872776
Fax: 01270 883556
E-mail: webmaster@raynauds.demon.co.uk
Website: <http://www.raynauds.demon.co.uk/>

Online discussion list
Name of list: **Scleroderma & Autoimmune Digest**

The scleroderma and autoimmune mailing list is intended to offer support to those who need it and educate each other as much as possible but most of all to show that many patients live well, and cope well with autoimmune disease. The list is also for the discussion of the latest research and practical clinical treatment guidelines in the disease area.

To join this discussion list send the following message:

To: sdandadigest-subscribe@egroups.com
Text: leave blank

Further information is available at: <http://sclerodermasupport.com/ support/digest/conditions.htm>

Online newsgroup
Name of newsgroup: <news://alt.support.scleroderma>

To view the Web archive of messages, go to <http://groups.google.com/> and enter the following: alt.support.scleroderma

Suggested summary documents

The US Arthritis Foundation provides a brief overview of scleroderma at: <http://www.arthritis.org/answers/diseasecenter/scleroderma.asp>.

The US Scleroderma Research Association also provides information in the form of 'facts' and 'symptoms' <http://www.srfcure.org/scleroderma.html>. It is also possible to join their mailing list by completing a secure form provided on the site.

Finally, the Mayo Clinic provides slightly more detailed information, including a description of two major forms of scleroderma. This can be found at: <http://www.mayoclinic.com/home?id=HQ01334>.

Scoliosis

Support group

Scoliosis Association (UK)
2 Ivebury Court
325 Latimer Road
London
W10 6RA

Tel: 020 8964 1166
Fax: 020 8964 5343
E-mail: info@sauk.org.uk
Web page: <http://www.sauk.org.uk/>

Online discussion list
Name of list: **SCOLIOSIS**

There are five related scoliosis mailing lists. Most subscribers prefer the digest – a single message sent out each day late at night (New York time) that groups all of the previous day's postings from all five lists: regular, medical, teens, parent, and child.

To join the digest, send the following message:

To: scoliosis-digest-request@ai.mit.edu
Text: subscribe

For more information, see
<http://www.ai.mit.edu/extra/scoliosis/scoliosis.html>.

Online newsgroup

At the time of writing, there was not a group devoted to scoliosis. However, the more general list <news://alt.support.chronic-pain> might be useful.

To view the Web archive of messages, go to <http://groups.google.com/> and enter the following: alt.support.chronic-pain

Suggested summary documents

The US Scoliosis Research Society provides an in-depth 'Review of scoliosis', which covers causes, diagnosis and treatment options for common types of spinal deformity. It can be found at:
<http://www.srs.org/htm/library/review/review00.htm>.

The Web site of the American Academy of Orthopedic Surgeons also provides a brief overview, available at:
<http://orthoinfo.aaos.org/brochure/thr_report.cfm?Thread_ID=14&topcategory=Spine>.

Further Internet-based scoliosis support groups and resources can be found at:
<http://www.ysabol.net/theinternetscoliosisclub/> and
<http://www.robsweb.karoo.net/scoliosis/>.

Seasonal affective disorder (SAD)

See also **Depression.**

Support group

SAD Association
PO Box 989
Steyning
West Sussex
BN44 3HG

Tel: 01903 814942
Fax: 01903 879939
E-mail: n/a
Web page: <http://www.sada.org.uk/>

Online discussion list

Name of list: **S-A-D**

For those suffering from seasonal affective disorder.

To join this discussion list send the following message:

To: S-A-D-subscribe@yahoogroups.com
Text: leave blank

Web archive of messages available at: <http://groups.yahoo.com/group/S-A-D>

Online newsgroup

Name of newsgroup: <news://alt.support.depression.seasonal>

To view the Web archive of messages, go to <http://groups.google.com/> and enter the following: alt.support.depression.seasonal

Suggested summary documents

The mental health charity Mind has produced a range of advice booklets giving straightforward practical information on a range of mental health issues. In recognition of their clarity, the booklets have won a Plain English Campaign Award. 'Understanding seasonal affective disorder' can be found at: <http://www.mind.org.uk/information/understanding/sad/understanding_seasonal_affective_disorder.asp>.

A short article on seasonal affective disorder and light therapy has been published by the National Institute for Medical Research. This paper discusses how light cycles and seasons could have a significant effect on moods and well being. It can be found at:
<http://www.nimr.mrc.ac.uk/MillHillEssays/1997/sad.htm>.

Sexually transmitted diseases

See also **Acquired Immune Deficiency Syndrome (AIDS)**

Support group

Family Planning Association
2–12 Pentonville Road
London N1 9FP

Tel: 0845 310 1334
Fax: 020 7837 3034
Web page: <http://www.fpa.org.uk/>

Online discussion list

Yahoo! Groups hosts over 40 groups classified under 'sexually transmitted diseases'. See:

<http://dir.groups.yahoo.com/dir/Health_Wellness/Support/Illnesses/ Sexually_Transmitted_Diseases_(STDs)>. Note that some of these groups have quite small memberships.

Online newsgroup

There is not a general list for discussion of sexually transmitted diseases, but there are groups for some specific conditions – for example: <news://alt.support.herpes>.

To view the Web archive of messages, go to <http://groups.google.com/> and enter the following: alt.support.herpes

Suggested summary documents

Lovelife <http://www.lovelife.uk.com/> is Health Promotion England's sexual health Web site. It provides up-to-date information on sexual health, including preventing and treating sexually transmitted diseases. The 'Check-up' section provides a list of addresses and opening times of sexual health clinics (sexually transmitted disease clinics) in the UK.

The US National Institute of Allergy and Infectious Diseases (NIAID) has produced a fact sheet entitled 'Introduction to sexually transmitted diseases'. It provides basic facts about sexually transmitted diseases, including the ways in which they are spread, their common symptoms, and how they can be treated. It can be found at: <http://www.niaid.nih.gov/factsheets/stdinfo.htm>.

The Men's Health Forum provides a brief overview called 'Sexually transmitted infections (STIs) and you'. It can be found at: <http://www. menshealthforum.org.uk/default.asp?goto=sexualhealth/index>. Alternatively, go to <http://www.menshealthforum.org.uk/> and click on the link 'Sexual Health'.

Sickle cell anaemia

Support group

Sickle Cell Society
54 Station Road
Harlesden
London
NW10 4UA

Tel: 020 8961 7795
Fax: 020 8961 8346
E-mail: sicklecellsoc@btinternet.com
Web page: <http://www.sicklecellsociety.org/>

Online discussion list
Name of list: **TheSickleCellForum**

'All are welcomed, whether you live with the disease, know someone who does or you're just curious.' Membership is at the discretion of the group moderators.

To join this discussion list send the following message:

To: TheSickleCellForum-subscribe@yahoogroups.com
Text: leave blank

Web archive of messages: for members only.

More information available at:
<http://groups.yahoo.com/group/TheSickleCellForum>

Online newsgroup
At the time of writing, there was not a group devoted to sickle cell anaemia. However, an analysis of postings that contain the words 'sickle cell anaemia' indicates that the newsgroup <news://misc.kids.info> frequently carries postings on this subject.

To view the Web archive of messages, go to <http://groups.google.com/> and enter the following: misc.kids.info

Suggested summary documents
The US National Heart, Lung, and Blood Institute has produced a fact sheet called 'Facts about sickle cell anemia'. It provides concise, accurate information on causes, populations affected, signs and symptoms, diagnoses and treatments. It is available in plain text format or as a PDF file (see Chapter 3) at:
<http://www.nhlbi.nih.gov/health/public/blood/sickle/sca_fact.htm>.

The Sickle Cell Information Centre
<http://www.emory.edu/PEDS/SICKLE/index.htm> has as its mission 'to provide sickle cell patient and professional education, news, research updates and world wide sickle cell resources'. All the content is reviewed by qualified physicians.

An article on sickle cell pain, produced by the Department of Pain Medicine and Palliative Care at Beth Israel Medical Centre, can be found at: <http://www.stoppain.org/education_research/SickleCellPain.html>.

Finally, Sickle Cell Online <http://member.aol.com/scd200/scd.htm> is a site 'dedicated to all Sickle Cell Sufferers in the United Kingdom and world-wide'.

Sleep disorders

Support groups
British Snoring and Sleep Apnoea Association
1 Duncroft Close
Reigate
Surrey
RH2 9DE

Tel: 0800 0851 097
Fax: 01737 248744
E-mail: snoreshop@britishsnoring.demon.co.uk
Web page: <http://www.britishsnoring.demon.co.uk>

Narcolepsy Association (UK)
1st Floor Craven House
121 Kingsway
London
WC2B 6PA

Tel: 020 7721 8904
Fax: 01322 863056
E-mail: info@narcolepsy.org.uk
Web page: <http://www.narcolepsy.org.uk/>

Online discussion list
Yahoo! Groups supports more than 20 discussion lists on sleep disorders, including insomnia, sleep apnoea, and restless leg syndrome – for a list, see: <http://dir.groups.yahoo.com/dir/Health_Wellness/Support/Illnesses/Sleep_Disorders>. Details of one of the more general lists are given below.

Name of list: **insomnia**

A list for sharing experiences of insomnia and suggesting remedies.

To join this discussion list send the following message:

To: insomnia-subscribe@yahoogroups.com
Text: leave blank

Web archive of messages available at:
<http://groups.yahoo.com/group/Insomnia>

Online newsgroup

Name of newsgroup: <news://alt.support.sleep-disorder>

To view the Web archive of messages, go to <http://groups.google.com/> and enter the following: alt.support.sleep-disorder

Suggested summary documents

The Royal College of Psychiatrists has produced a leaflet called 'Sleeping well'. It describes some common problems in both children and adults; provides simple guidelines to help with better sleep; and offers advice about deciding when to ask for professional help. Subjects include narcolepsy, sleep apnoea, sleepwalking, night terrors, nightmares and restless legs. It can be found at: <http://www.rcpsych.ac.uk/public/help/sleep/index.htm>.

The Sleep Council is funded by the UK bed industry but offers impartial advice. Tips for sleep can be found at <http://www.sleepcouncil.org.uk/>.

Stomach cancer

See also **Cancer.**

Support group

There is not a UK support group specifically for stomach cancer, but there are several cancer support groups, for example:

CancerBACUP
3 Bath Place
Rivington Street
London
EC2A 3JR

Tel (Helpline): 0808 800 1234
Tel: 020 7696 9003
Fax: 020 7696 9002
E-mail: info@cancerbacup.org
Web page: <http://www.cancerbacup.org.uk/>

Online discussion list
Name of list: **STOMACH-ONC**

STOMACH-ONC is an unmoderated discussion list for patients, family, friends, researchers, and physicians, to discuss clinical and non-clinical issues and advances relating to stomach and gastric cancer.

To join this discussion list send the following message:

To: listserv@listserv.acor.org
Text: subscribe stomach-onc

Web archive of messages available at: <http://listserv.acor.org/archives/stomach-onc.html>

Online newsgroup
Name of newsgroup: <news://alt.support.cancer>

To view the Web archive of messages, go to <http://groups.google.com/> and enter the following: alt.support.cancer

Suggested summary documents
As part of its excellent booklet series, the charity Cancer BACUP has produced 'Understanding cancer of the stomach'. As well as explaining causes, symptoms, diagnosis and treatment, it discusses the emotional shock of a cancer diagnosis, and provides information about useful organisations and 'recommended reading'. It can be found at:
<http://www.cancerbacup.org.uk/info/stomach.htm>.

The US National Cancer Institute provides a clear and informative overview called 'What you need to know about cancer of the stomach'. This is available at: <http://cancernet.nci.nih.gov/wyntk_pubs/stomach.htm>.

Stress

Support groups
First Steps to Freedom
7 Avon Court
School Lane
Kenilworth
Warwickshire
CV8 2GX

Tel: 01926 851608
Fax: 01926 864473
E-mail: info@firststeps.demon.co.uk
Web page: <http://www.firststeps.demon.co.uk/>

'Unwind' (Pain and Stress Management)
Melrose
3 Alderlea Close
Gilesgate
Durham
DH1 1DS
Tel/fax: 0191 384 2056

Online discussion list
Yahoo! Groups hosts over 40 groups classified under 'stress management' – see <http://dir.groups.yahoo.com/dir/Health_Wellness/Stress_Management>.

Online newsgroup
Name of newsgroup: <news://alt.support.anxiety-panic>

To view the Web archive of messages, go to <http://groups.google.com/> and enter the following: alt.support.anxiety-panic

Suggested summary documents
The American Psychological Association has produced a set of documents collected under the title 'Focus on Stress'. Specific titles include 'How does stress affect us?', 'Stress in the workplace' and the 'Road to burnout'. They can be found at <http://helping.apa.org/work/>.

Northumberland Mental Health Trust has produced a range of free online self-help guides. They can be viewed at: <http://www.northumberland-haz.org.uk/selfhelp/default.htm>.

Relax4free <http://www.relax4free.co.uk/index.htm> is a site provided by Stress Control UK 'dedicated to combating the effects of stress and anxiety'.

Stroke

Support group
Stroke Association
123–127 Whitecross Street
London
EC1Y 8JJ

Tel: 0845 3033 100
Fax: 020 7490 2686
E-mail: stroke@stroke.org.uk
Web page: <http://www.stroke.org.uk/>

Online discussion list

Name of list: **strokesurvivors**

An online international stroke support group.

To join this discussion list send the following message:

To: strokesurvivors-subscribe@yahoogroups.com
Text: leave blank

Web archive of messages: for members only.

More information available at: <http://groups.yahoo.com/group/strokesurvivors> and <http://strokesurvivors.org>

Online newsgroup

There is not a group specifically about stroke, but it has been discussed in various groups, in particular <news://alt.support.disorders.neurological>.

To view the Web archive of messages, go to <http://groups.google.com/> and enter the following: alt.support.disorders.neurological

Suggested summary documents

The US National Institute of Neurological Disorders and Stroke has produced a detailed online guide called 'Stroke: hope through research'. Particular attention is given to risk factors. It can be found at: <http://www.ninds.nih.gov/health_and_medical/pubs/stroke_hope_through_research.htm>.

BBC Health hosts a stroke guide Web site at: <http://www.bbc.co.uk/health/stroke/>. Topics covered include causes, symptoms, treatment, rehabilitation and prevention.

Different Strokes <http://www.differentstrokes.co.uk/> is a UK charity set up 'by younger stroke survivors for younger stroke survivors, for the purposes of active self-help and mutual support'.

Sudden infant death syndrome (SIDS)

Support groups

Foundation for the Study of Infant Deaths
Artillery House
11–19 Artillery Row
London
SW1P 1RT

Tel: 020 7233 2090
Fax: 020 7222 8002
E-mail: fsid@sids.org.uk
Web page: <http://www.sids.org.uk/fsid/>

Cot Death Society
Units 6 & 8
Padgate Business Centre
Green Lane
Warrington
WA1 4JN

Tel: 0845 6010234
Fax: 01925 851943
E-mail: fundraising@cotdeathsociety.org.uk
Web page: <http://www.cotdeathsociety.org.uk/>

Online discussion list

Name of list: **sidslist**

Sidslist is intended to provide a safe, secure environment for individuals seeking support after losing a child to SIDS (Sudden infant death syndrome).

To join this discussion list send the following message:

To: sidslist-subscribe@yahoogroups.com
Text: leave blank

Web archive of messages: for members only.

More information available at: <http://groups.yahoo.com/group/sidslist>

Online newsgroup

Name of newsgroup: <news://alt.support.grief>

To view the Web archive of messages, go to <http://groups.google.com/> and enter the following: alt.support.grief

Suggested summary documents

The Foundation for the Study of Infant Deaths provides information on cot death at: <http://www.sids.org.uk/fsid/cot.htm>. It includes advice on reducing the risk of cot death.

The Department of Health has produced a leaflet called 'Reduce the risk of cot death: an easy guide', available at: <http://www.doh.gov.uk/cotdeath/index.htm>.

Testicular cancer

See also **Cancer.**

Support group

Wessex Cancer Trust Helpline for Men with Cancer
Bellis House
11 Westwood Road
Southampton
Hampshire
SO17 1DL

Tel: 023 8067 2200
Fax: 023 8067 2266
E-mail: wct@wessexcancer.org
Web page: <http://www.wessexcancer.org/>

Online discussion list

Name of list: **TC-NET: The Testicular Cancer Online Support Group**

TC-NET is an unmoderated discussion list for patients, family, friends, researchers and physicians, to discuss clinical and non-clinical issues and advances relating to testicular cancer.

To join this discussion list send the following message:

To: listserv@listserv.acor.org
Text: subscribe tc-net

Web archive of messages available at: <http://listserv.acor.org/archives/tc-net.html>

Online newsgroup

Name of newsgroup: <news://alt.support.cancer.testicular>

To view the Web archive of messages, go to <http://groups.google.com/> and enter the following: alt.support.cancer.testicular

Suggested summary documents

As part of its excellent booklet series, the charity Cancer BACUP has produced 'Understanding testicular cancer'. As well as explaining causes, symptoms, diagnosis and treatment, it discusses the emotional shock of a cancer diagnosis and provides information about useful organisations and 'recommended reading'. It can be found at:
<http://www.cancerbacup.org.uk/info/testes.htm>.

The Imperial Cancer Research Fund runs the 'Everyman' campaign to raise awareness of male cancers (particularly testicular and prostate cancer) and to raise funds to build the UK's first dedicated male cancer research centre. More information can be found at: <http://www.icr.ac.uk/everyman/>. A 'Testicular cancer fact sheet' provides a brief overview, and includes an illustrated guide to self-examination. It is available at:
<http://www.icr.ac.uk/everyman/about/testicular.html>.

Throat, cancer of

See **Oral cancer.**

Thyroid cancer

See also **Cancer.**

Support group

There is not a UK support group specifically for thyroid cancer, but there are several cancer support groups, for example:

CancerBACUP
3 Bath Place
Rivington Street
London
EC2A 3JR

Tel: 0808 800 1234
Fax: 020 7696 9002
E-mail: info@cancerbacup.org
Web page: <http://www.cancerbacup.org.uk/>

Online discussion list

Name of list: **THYROID-ONC (The Thyroid Cancer Online Support Group)**

THYROID-ONC is an unmoderated discussion list for patients, family, friends, researchers and physicians, to discuss clinical and non-clinical issues and advances relating to thyroid cancer.

To join this discussion list send the following message:

To: listserv@listserv.acor.org
Text: subscribe thyroid-onc

Web archive of messages available at: <http://listserv.acor.org/archives/thyroid-onc.html>

Online newsgroups

Name of newsgroup: <news://alt.support.thyroid>
Name of newsgroup: <news://alt.support.cancer>

To view the Web archives of messages, go to <http://groups.google.com/> and enter either: alt.support.thyroid *or* alt.support.cancer

Suggested summary documents

As part of its excellent booklet series, the charity Cancer BACUP has produced 'Understanding cancer of the thyroid'. As well as explaining causes, symptoms, diagnosis and treatment, it discusses the emotional shock of a cancer diagnosis, and provides information about useful organisations and 'recommended reading'. It can be found at: <http://www.cancerbacup.org.uk/info/thyroid.htm>.

The US National Cancer Institute provides an overview in the form of 'Questions and answers about thyroid cancer' at: <http://cis.nci.nih.gov/fact/6_31.htm>.

Tinnitus

Support group

Royal National Institute for Deaf People (RNID)
19–23 Featherstone Street
London
EC1Y 8SL

Tel: 0808 808 0123
Fax: 020 7296 8199
E-mail: helpline@rnid.org.uk
Web page: <http://www.rnid.org.uk/>

Online discussion list

Name of list: **our-ears**

A list for people who are suffering from hearing loss and hearing disorders, including Ménière's disease, tinnitus, sensineural hearing loss, and profound hearing losses. 'We welcome people who are hearing, hard of hearing and deaf joining together in support and friendship in a comfortable forum while learning about their disorders and overcoming difficulties and the symptoms associated with them.'

To join this discussion list send the following message:

To: our-ears-subscribe@yahoogroups.com
Text: leave blank

Web archive of messages: for members only.

More information available at: <http://groups.yahoo.com/group/our-ears>

Online newsgroup

Name of newsgroup: <news://alt.support.tinnitus>

To view the Web archive of messages, go to <http://groups.google.com/> and enter the following: alt.support.tinnitus

Suggested summary documents

The RNID provides clear and detailed information about tinnitus on its Web site, with an information page at <http://www.rnid.org.uk/html/info_tinnitus.htm>. It includes a link to a list of fact sheets on many aspects of the condition. About half of them are available online, and the rest can be ordered by completing a form (free for single copies for private use).

Two UK charities, Tinnitus Action and Action for Tinnitus Research, share a news page at <http://www.tinnitus-research.org/frameset.html>. It includes a link to the current issue of 'SOUND*Sense*', a quarterly journal that 'offers practical help in dealing with the burden or annoyance of tinnitus'.

Tourette syndrome

Support group
Tourette Syndrome (UK) Association
The Administration Office
Old Grange House
The Twitten
Southview Road
Crowborough
East Sussex
TN6 1HF

Tel: 01892 669151 (voicemail/fax)
E-mail: enquiries@tsa.org.uk
Web page: <http://www.tsa.org.uk/>

Online discussion list
Name of list: **tourette**

Support group for parents of children diagnosed with Tourette syndrome.

To join this discussion list send the following message:

To: tourette-subscribe@yahoogroups.com
Text: leave blank

Web archive of messages: for members only.

More information available at: <http://groups.yahoo.com/group/tourette>

Online newsgroup
Name of newsgroup: <news://alt.support.tourette>

To view the Web archive of messages, go to <http://groups.google.com/> and enter the following: alt.support.tourette

Suggested summary documents
The US National Institute of Neurological Disorders and Stroke has produced a 'Tourette syndrome fact sheet'. It provides a clear overview, covering symptoms diagnosis, treatment and prognosis – see: <http://www.ninds.nih.gov/health_and_medical/pubs/tourette_syndrome.htm>.

Tourette Syndrome Support in the UK <http://www.tourettesyndrome.co.uk/> is a page produced by 'a mum who wanted to provide some info about TS in the UK'. It provides an extensive range of information and support, including links to other sites.

Tuberculosis

Support group
Breathe Easy Club
British Lung Foundation
78 Hatton Garden
London
EC1N 8JR

Tel: 020 7831 5831
Fax: 020 7831 5832
E-mail: breatheasy@britishlungfoundation.com
Web page: <http://www.lunguk.org/index.html>

Online discussion list
Name of list: **tbnet**

The purpose of the tbnet e-mail list is to provide a forum for exchange of information and discussion on matters relating to tuberculosis (TB). The e-mail list is open to all and moderated, and currently has 540 subscribers in 64 countries.

To join this discussion list send the following message:

To: majordomo@mos.com.np
Text: subscribe tbnet

Web archive of messages: not available.

More information can be found at: <http://www.tb.net.np/e-mail.html>

Online newsgroup
Name of newsgroup: <news:alt.support.tuberculosis>

To view the Web archive of messages, go to <http://groups.google.com/> and enter the following: alt.support.tuberculosis

Suggested summary documents
The TB Network Web site, which was launched on 24 March 2000, World TB Day, aims to 'provide support and information for anyone affected by, or

infected with, TB'. A section called 'TB answers' provides an overview of the condition in the form of questions and answers, whilst 'Medical info' provides information about drug treatments. Other sections cover news, personal stories, and book reviews. The site can be accessed at: <http://www.tbnet-work.co.uk/>.

The American Lung Association also uses the question and answer format to provide information on symptoms, diagnosis and treatment – see: <http://www.lungusa.org/diseases/lungtb.html>.

Urinary tract infections

Support group
National Kidney Federation
6 Stanley Street
Worksop
England
S81 7HX

Tel: 0845 6010209
Fax: 01909 481723
E-mail: mks@kidney.org.uk
Web page: <http://www.kidney.org.uk/>

Online discussion list
Name of list: **kidneydis**

A list for those living with various chronic kidney/urinary tract diseases to discuss causes, manifestations, treatments, side effects and coping strategies.

To join this discussion list send the following message:

To: kidneydis-subscribe@yahoogroups.com
Text: leave blank

Web archive of messages: for members only.

For more information, see: <http://groups.yahoo.com/group/kidneydis>.

Online newsgroup
There is no group devoted to urinary tract infections, but it has been discussed in the <news://sci.med.prostate.prostatitis> group.

Name of newsgroup: <news://sci.med.prostate.prostatitis>

To view the Web archive of messages, go to <http://groups.google.com/> and enter the following: sci.med.prostate.prostatitis

Suggested summary documents

The US National Institute of Diabetes and Digestive and Kidney Diseases (NIDDK) has produced an online patient information leaflet called 'Urinary tract infection in adults', which looks at causes, risk factors, symptoms and treatment. It is available at:
<http://www.niddk.nih.gov/health/urolog/pubs/utiadult/utiadult.htm>.

The American Foundation for Urologic Disease provides a brief but clear overview at <http://www.afud.org/conditions/uti.html>. It includes diagrams of the male and female urinary systems, and also lists conditions that may be confused with urinary tract infections.

Varicose veins

Support group
British Vascular Foundation
Griffin House
West Street
Woking
GU21 1EB

Tel: 01483 726511
Fax: 01483 726522
E-mail: bvf@care4free.net
Web page: <http://www.bvf.org.uk/>

Online discussion list
Name of list: **VaricoseVeinsSupport**

A list for people who suffer from varicose veins and would like to talk to others with the same problem. (Note: it has quite a small membership, and a low volume of mails.)

To join this discussion list send the following message:

To: varicoseveinssupport-subscribe@yahoogroups.com
Text: leave blank

Web archive of messages available at:
<http://groups.yahoo.com/group/VaricoseVeinsSupport>

Online newsgroup
There is no group specifically about varicose veins but the subject has been discussed in a variety of groups, in particular <news://misc.kids.pregnancy>.

To view the Web archive of messages, go to <http://groups.google.com/> and enter the following: misc.kids.pregnancy

Suggested summary documents

The Veins Website <http://www.veins.co.uk/> is written by Mr Mark Whiteley, a Consultant Vascular Surgeon and Visiting Senior Fellow in Vascular Surgery at the University of Surrey. The site includes a section called 'Myths about veins'.

The British Vascular Foundation provides a brief overview in the form of questions and answers. It can be found at: <http://www.bvf.org.uk/new_page_11.htm#Your Varicose Veins Questions Answered>.

Index